JUICE IT!
BLEND IT!

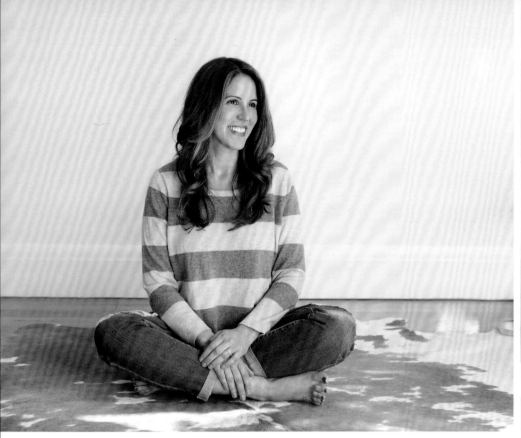
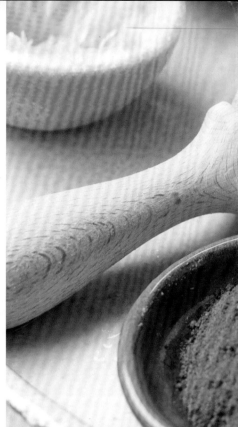

Lisa Craven is a juice devotee from New York City. She developed her passion for juicing eight years ago when, at a friend's apartment in New York City, she decided she needed a wine-free night and instead tried a green juice. She never looked back. Lisa is passionate about wellbeing and keeping life in balance. Her passion is for everyone to juice and live long, healthy and balanced lives.

In addition to daily juicing she has created a fabulous life filled with yoga, meditation, affirmations and healthy people around her. She has over fifteen years of experience in Human Resources and Talent where she has focused on keeping employees healthy and well balanced at work. She went through intense yoga teacher training, is a Life and Executive Coach and a champion for wellness in the workplace. She has found true reward in helping those who want a life filled with wellness in Sydney where she now resides.

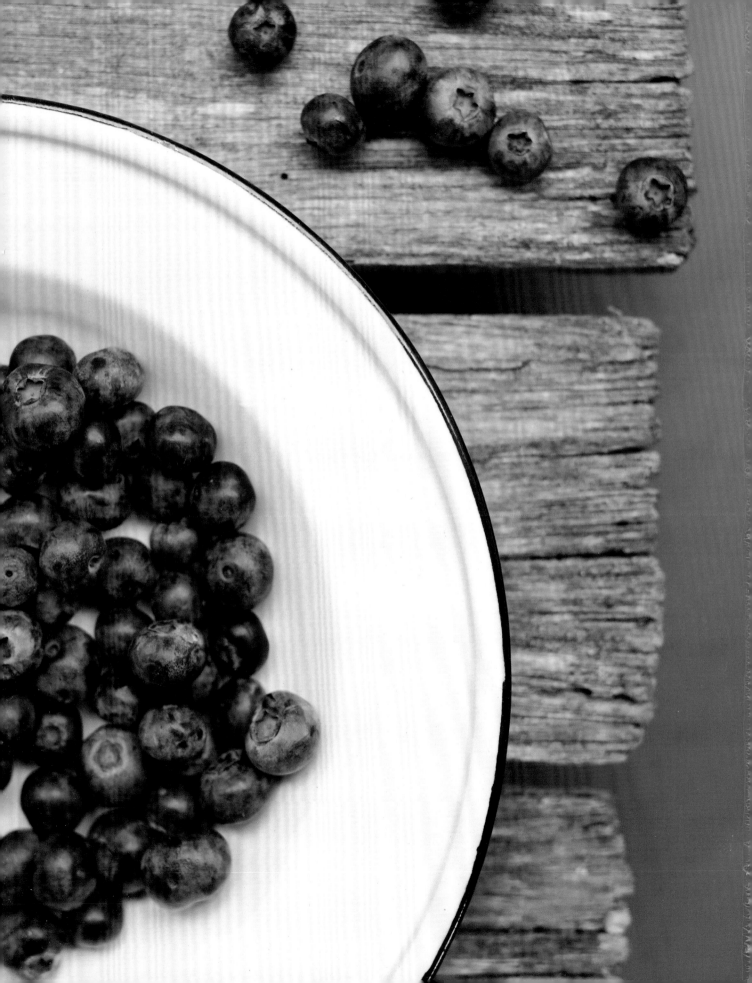

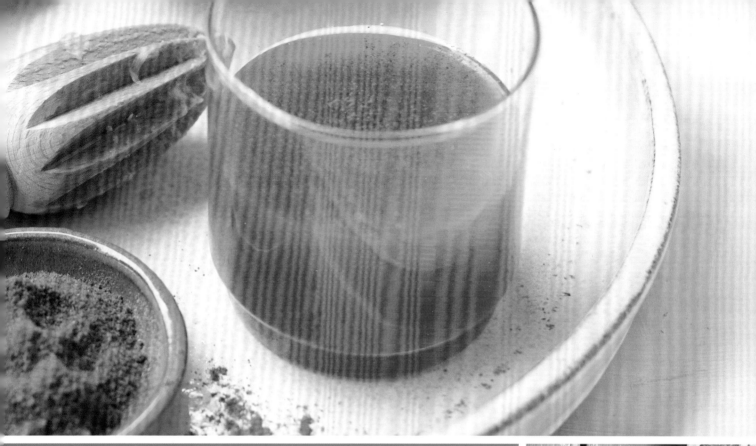

JUICE IT!
BLEND IT!

TRANSFORM YOUR HEALTH ONE DRINK AT A TIME!

LISA CRAVEN

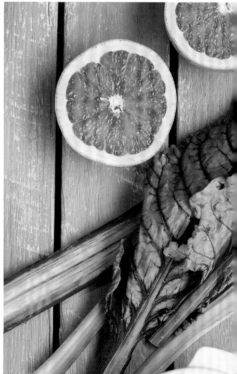

First published 2015

Exisle Publishing Pty Ltd
'Moonrising', Narone Creek Road, Wollombi,
NSW 2325, Australia
P.O. Box 60–490, Titirangi, Auckland 0642,
New Zealand
www.exislepublishing.com

A CiP record for this book is available from the
National Library of Australia.

ISBN 978 1 921966 80 4

Design and typesetting by Tracey Gibbs
Photographs by Bayleigh Vedegalo
Juice styling by Rhianne Contreras
Typeset in Hurme Geometric Sans
Printed in China

This book uses paper sourced under ISO 14001
guidelines from well-managed forests and other
controlled sources.

10 9 8 7 6 5 4 3 2 1

Disclaimer
While this book is intended as a general information
resource and all care has been taken in compiling
the contents, this book does not take account of
individual circumstances and is not a substitute for
medical advice. Always consult a qualified practitioner
or therapist. Neither the author nor the publisher and
their distributors can be held responsible for any loss,
claim or action that may arise from reliance on the
information contained in this book.

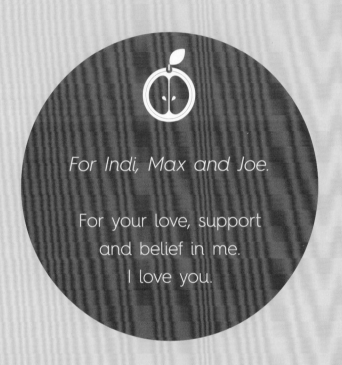

For Indi, Max and Joe.

For your love, support
and belief in me.
I love you.

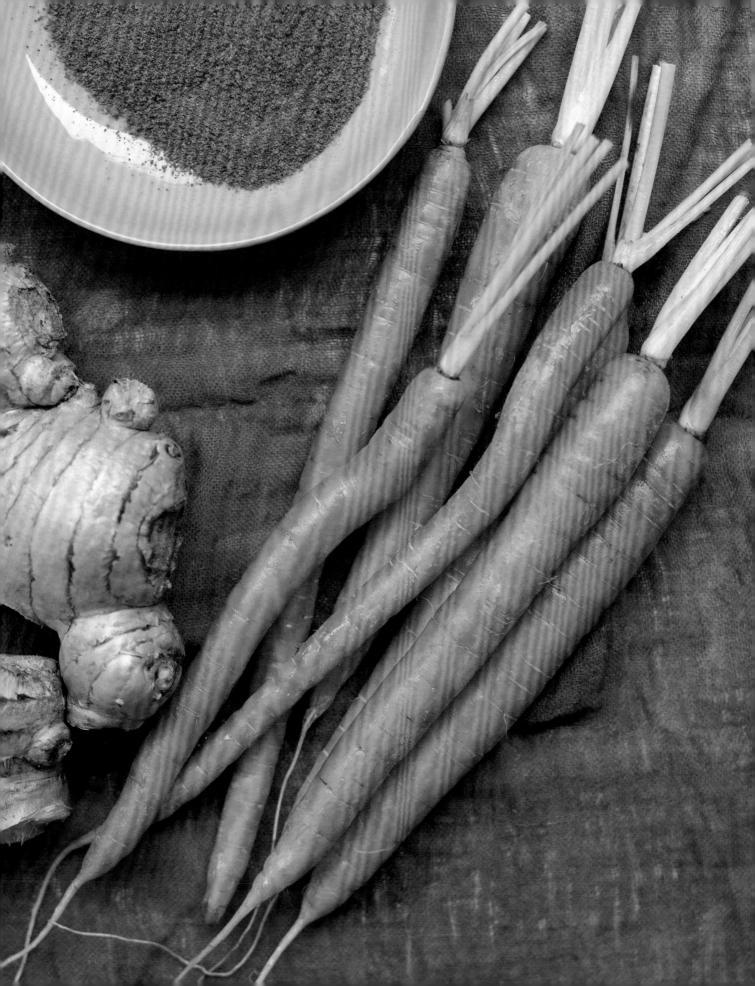

CONTENTS

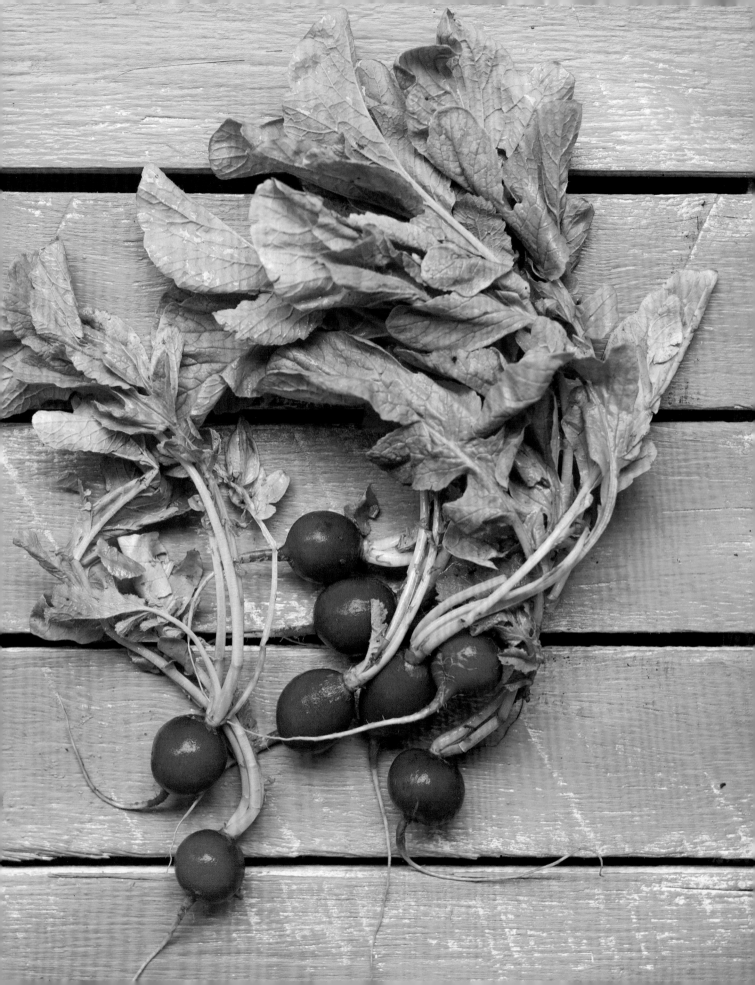

WELLNESS, BEAUTY & WISDOM

A LITTLE ABOUT ME

I am a woman who is passionate about wellbeing, balance, yoga and positive thinking. As much as I strive for this daily, life sometimes gets in the way and throws me a curve ball. The pressures and struggles of life happen, and I always find myself trying to get back on the path to wellness, wisdom and beauty. My journey has encouraged me to be who I am today, and has shown me that sometimes you have to hit rock bottom before you can pick up the pieces and get back up. Rock bottom is the place where I learned to take care of myself, to look after my health and find the balance that is the key to staying well.

About eight years ago I went through a period in my life where I felt continually sick, tired and stressed. The only way I knew how to get to work every day and maintain a fun social life was to drink too much coffee and keep going and going. I picked up take-away food, I drank loads of bubbly champagne, and I let sleep drop away as a priority. I was living in New York City — the city that never ever sleeps — enjoying life on the go, but my health was suffering and I didn't understand why.

Eventually I found an amazing chiropractor who helped get me back on track. She made me realize that in order to feel, look and be my best I needed to understand what was really going on inside my body. This started with my diet. *Diet?*, I thought … *Well, I eat when I'm hungry, and my work, travel and social plans mean that often involves eating out or on the go.* My chiro asked me to keep a food diary. My heart sank. A food diary? I came back a week later, ashamed of myself. For the first time in my life I recognized that I wasn't looking after my health; indeed, I was completely neglecting it. After a closer look at what I was — and, importantly, what I wasn't — eating I knew that it was time to take control of my health before it took control of me. I just needed to learn how.

I think of that New York chiro all the time. She ran blood tests and explained I had vitamin deficiencies that could be cleared up with diet. She told me I was gluten intolerant, yet without celiac disease. She explained what I needed to eat and how to incorporate food and juice into my diet to make sure I got the nutrients I needed. She sat with me for hours on end explaining how to change my life and regain control of my health.

I thought I had been looking after myself, but just giving up the bubbly wasn't going to cut it. I had to do something severe to regain my health and wellbeing, and it began with a three-week deep cleanse. This, of course, meant cutting out alcohol, dairy, meat, gluten, sugar and caffeine (the hardest for me), along with taking adequate time to rest and heal. Lots of water, lots of lemon and my kitchen was exploding in everything green. My new morning routine consisted of getting up early to breathe and stretch, followed by a full day of smoothies and some raw foods. I consumed six liquid or raw meals, I didn't skip meals and I planned ahead. No heavy exercise, just walking and clearing my mind. I will confess that these three weeks took me on an emotional rollercoaster. As my body went through these changes my mind tried to tell me I was doing more harm than good — and that champagne and bagels were the best things for me. I was angry and irritable from a lack of protein. I felt deprived of a social life, as smoothies aren't exactly served at the local bar. However, I carried on with my plan, pushing through to prove to myself I could do it. Towards the end of the cleanse I noticed changes: I felt full of life and clear-headed.

I quickly became hooked on feeling good. My body and I became friends as my thoughts, habits and views on wellness changed. The dinners-on-the-go went, and checking ingredients and maintaining balance became part of my life.

I thought I had become a super health nut, but it wasn't until I visited the home of a close friend that my life truly changed. She raved about her juicer and showed me her refrigerator, which was filled with more greens than I could pronounce. She was what I would call a juice fanatic, and it is because of her that I discovered the power of juicing. Until then I'd had no desire to drink that many vegetables in a day; I didn't even know what a juicer was or how it worked.

The short story here is that one day I tried a green juice and never looked back. I loved it. Instead of champagne and a cheese board on a Friday evening, I started to opt for fresh homemade green juices. Even I was surprised. How could vegetables taste so good that I craved them? How was it that I now looked at spinach with love and craved kale on Friday nights? Smoothies became a sweet obsession. They are delicious tasting, nutritious and loaded with goodness that gave me more sustained energy than a blueberry muffin or cappuccino.

I was hooked — on juicing my vegetables for the taste and the nutrition value, and on my new smoothies that tasted better than desserts. I was so hooked I joined a local food co-operative in Brooklyn, one of the largest food co-ops in the United States, and it gave me access to organic, locally grown fruit and vegetables. I was on a track to health, and this is where all the fun began.

I started to experiment, playing with different combinations in my juicer and blender, knowing that everything I put in it could help my body heal more than any pill ever could. I found myself buying vegetables I had never cooked before and trying them in my juicer — and the rest is history.

I am no longer sick. I am no longer tired. I now feel great. My skin glows. My juices and smoothies are full of vitamins and minerals that help me stay healthy. My body cleanses itself on a daily basis. Juicing has become part of my life.

SO, WHY *JUICE IT! BLEND IT!?*

In the context of health, has anyone ever told you that you should eat more cheese, load up on bread, or have another rib-eye steak? Have you ever been told to drink more beer or wine? What about eating more vegetables? You got it. Since we were little we have been told to eat our vegetables, even though we probably didn't really understand why — only that vegetables were good for us. As adults, though, we know that incorporating vegetables into our daily diet is necessary to keep us free from disease. According to World Health Organization dietary guidelines we should all be increasing our vegetable intake, which in turn means decreasing our chance of becoming obese or overweight, and of developing cancer, cardiovascular disease, stroke and many other diseases. There are only advantages to having your daily dose of vegetables.

We may know the benefits of eating our fruit and vegetables, but incorporating them into our diet is tricky, and can sometimes seem impossible when we lead a busy life. We often eat on the run — as I used to do — or make meals that are quick and easy, which often can be unhealthy and lacking in nutrients. This is where it all goes wrong. Our body and mind suffer as we fill them with artificial, chemical-filled foods and sweeteners, leaving us feeling sick and tired. In turn, we start to crave more 'junk' food and sweet 'treats' and we end up with health issues we can't understand. Even if we manage to find a doctor or naturopath who will prescribe us something or offer suggestions on natural remedies, we still can't seem to squeeze health and deliciousness back into our lives.

Does this sound familiar to you? If it does, let me assure you of something: you're not alone. We all go through what feel like normal times, calm times and then hectic times where things move so fast we prioritize work and all the things that seem more important than looking after our health.

If you want to prevent or recover from illness, or stay healthy, or lose weight and/or increase energy, then juicing is for you. *Juice It! Blend It!* is a juice reference guide that will show you how to incorporate plant foods into your everyday diet. It will help you to live a healthy, happy life with one simple juice a day. In eight chapters full of information and support I review the six Ws of juicing:

> » **Who should juice.**
> » **What you should put in your juice.**
> » **Where you should juice.**
> » **When you should juice.**
> » **Why you should juice.**
> » **Which type of juicer or blender you need.**

Each chapter focuses on the benefits and ease of juicing, along with facts and fun tidbits from a wellness nut who loves to juice and blend plant food. Included are yummy recipes for anyone and everyone as well as disease-fighting power juices for those who want to self-heal. The benefits of juicing are endless, and this book will show you that one simple juice a day can add years to your life.

Tip: LIVE A LIFE IN BALANCE. ONE FRESH VEGETABLE JUICE A DAY AND YOU CAN BE LIVING A FULLER, RICHER, HEALTHIER, LONGER LIFE.

WHAT ARE THE HEALTH BENEFITS OF JUICING?

Juices are packed with fruit and vegetables, giving you the goodness you need from vitamins, minerals and enzymes. According to the World Cancer Research Fund we should be eating 600 grams — at least five servings — of fruits and vegetables per day, from a wide range of colours for maximum nutritional impact. How will you manage to eat twelve carrots today? You will juice them! You can meet your daily needs simply through juicing. The bottom line is to eat your vegetables and mix them up. Packing different vegetables in your juice each day will give you the energy your body needs and craves.

So, what's all the hype about vegetables? Vegetables are an excellent source of vitamins and minerals. They help build a strong immune system, protect us from disease, and are full of antioxidants and vitamins such as Vitamin A, B, C, E and magnesium. They give us all the nutrients we need to keep us healthy and help our bodies be proactive in avoiding illness, including the scary Cs: cancer, cardiovascular disease and corpulence (obesity). (According to the Harvard School of Public Health, 35 per cent of all cancer deaths are potentially avoidable by dietary change.) There are only benefits to increasing our daily diet of vegetables, which in turn adds vitamins to our diet in the form of food. Vitamins in the form of a capsule won't give the same effect as juicing, which gets into the bloodstream within twenty minutes.

The benefits are endless. You aren't too busy to juice or blend. You can still eat out, too. This book contains more than 100 easy recipes that will help you incorporate juicing into your already busy life.

To a life of wellness, beauty and wisdom, *Lisa x*

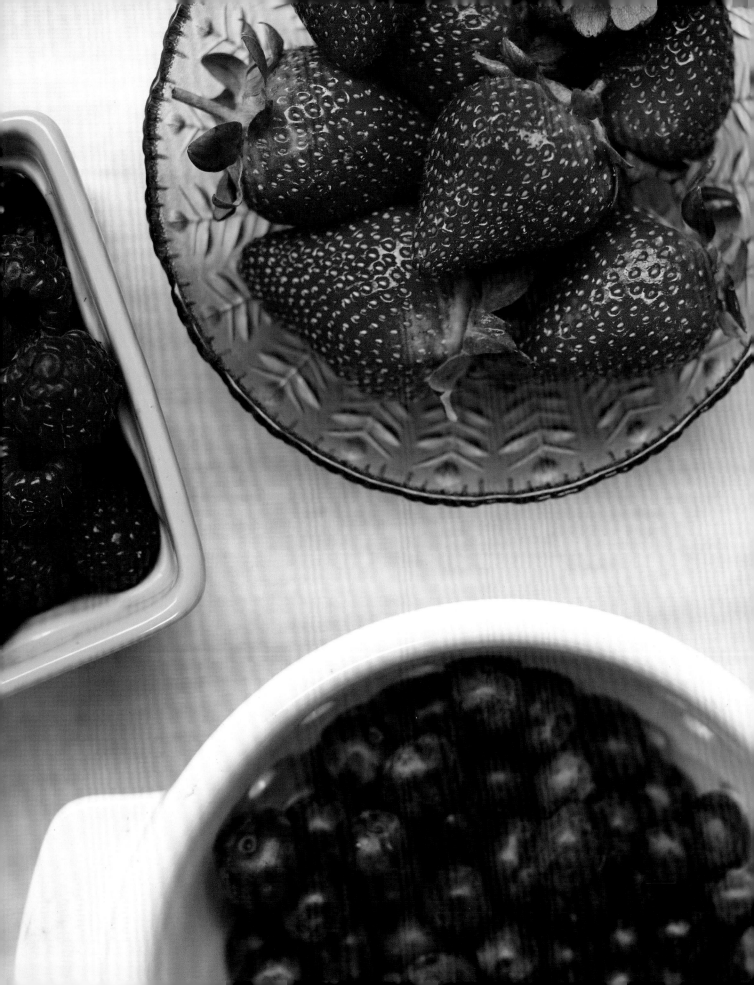

CHAPTER 1

EVERYTHING JUICY

There are so many benefits to juicing, and so many questions to ask and choices to make. For starters, you might be thinking: Should I juice or blend? Which juicer should I buy? Do I need a blender? What about kale versus spinach? Should I freeze my bananas to make my smoothie thicker and creamier? How do I add superfoods to my juices and smoothies? Wait, I want to make nut milk — how can I do this at home? Someone mentioned alkaline levels and I have no idea what they are talking about. Everyone is drinking coconut water, and not just on the beach — why?

Discover how amazing your life can be with just one smoothie or juice a day!

You get my point. There is so much information out there, so my aim in this book is to give you a taste of how amazing your life will be after you incorporate a juice or smoothie each day. In this chapter I will guide you through the process of getting started, choosing the right equipment, compiling the right tools in your kitchen and gathering the right ingredients, along with answering your questions about where, when and how you can juice and blend every day with ease.

JUICING OR BLENDING AT HOME VERSUS BUYING

'So, what's all the fuss about? I'll just buy my juice at the supermarket,' is what I have heard before. NO! People have asked me why they should go through all of this trouble — buying a juicer and all the ingredients — when they can simply buy a juice or smoothie at the local grocery store. I always tell them that juicing and blending best takes place at home, and here is why:

> » **Sugar — juices you buy off a shelf are usually loaded with sugar and lack nutrients.**
>
> » **Pasteurization — pre-packaged juices need a shelf life so manufacturers use a process of heating to kill bacteria, but this takes the nutrients with it.**
>
> » **Preservatives — ditto for preservatives; they are what give pre-packaged juices their store shelf life.**
>
> » **Expense — juicing and blending at home is not only better for you, but will save you money over the long term.**

JUICING VERSUS BLENDING: IS THERE A DIFFERENCE?

The short answer is: yes. They use different equipment, they taste different, and they have different consistencies and different health benefits.

Juicing contains no fibre, allowing vitamins and minerals to immediately be absorbed into the body and give you an instant energy boost.

On the other hand, blending — or smoothie-making — is full of fibre, takes longer for the body to absorb the nutrients and is equivalent to a meal replacement. Basically, you can have many juices in one day, but a single smoothie will fill you up.

Juicing happens in a machine that does the work for you, mechanically separating the liquid from the solid or pulp of the fruit or vegetable, leaving the indigestible fibre behind. This means that juices are easier than smoothies to digest. Once the pulp is discarded, you can use it in many different ways, including my top three: compost it; give it to your neighbour's chickens; or cook and bake with it.

Blending, or smoothie-making, keeps everything intact, including the fibre. Blending takes place in a blender and requires greater preparation, including peeling, pitting and cutting the fruit and vegetables, and then adding liquid, which keeps all the yummy flavour and texture.

Let's recap. The main differences between juicing and blending are:

JUICING

» The result is a juice, which gives you energy through a quick (within twenty minutes) absorption of vitamins, minerals and enzymes into your bloodstream.

» Your digestive system doesn't have to work hard.

» Juicing separates the pulp from the juice.

» Juice keeps you hydrated.

» Juice does not contain fibre.

» Juicing uses vegetables, and some fruit.

» Vegetable preparation is easy (small pieces are required for some juicers, but you won't need to peel).

» Fruit and vegetables need to be cleaned to remove pesticides.

» You won't feel full after a juice; it's not a meal replacement except when you are doing a cleanse.

BLENDING

» The result is a smoothie, which gives you that full feeling; a smoothie can be a snack or a meal.

» Blending requires digestion because it retains the fibre of the fruit and/or vegetable.

» Blending leaves pulp in the smoothie.

» Fruit and vegetables need to be cleaned to remove pesticides.

» Sugars in fruit absorb more slowly than with juiced vegetables.

» You can add protein powders and healthy yummy fats such as avocado to a smoothie.

» Blending uses fruits, including bananas, avocados, thick fruits and leafy vegetables.

» You can add many fun ingredients, such as nuts, nut butters, liquid and ice.

SHOULD I JUICE OR BLEND?

Do both, but at different times during the day. A juice is a great addition to a meal, but a smoothie can be the meal in itself. Just keep in mind that the ingredients, preparation and recipes are different and not always interchangeable. You can also juice vegetables and add them to your smoothie instead of another liquid, giving you the best of both worlds. For example, make a mean green juice (see recipe on page 26) and then add that to your smoothie — and *voilà!*, you have a nutritious blend of juice and smoothie. This is delicious, healthy and requires both a juicer and a blender.

Juicing is an easy way to add vegetables to your diet.

Some people will use a blender and a juicer. I do. They each serve a different purpose, almost like a toaster and a microwave — both heat up food, but the outcome of the food as well as the taste and texture are different. It's great if you can have both a juicer and blender, but that's not everyone's cup of tea. If you can only choose one, my suggestion is to go with a juicer if you are looking to add vegetables to your diet and want the vegetables to be assimilated quickly, giving you loads of energy. However, a note about juicing fruit: if you plan to juice a lot of fruit be careful, because this can cause a rapid spike in blood sugar, which often leads to energy loss rather than gain. If you are looking for extra yummy fibre with slow absorption of food and a snack or meal replacement, go with a blender.

WHAT FRUITS AND VEGETABLES CAN BE JUICED OR BLENDED?

Here is a simple way to remember. Vegetables, and some fruit, that are high in water content go in the juicer. Fruit and vegetables with very little water content — such as bananas or avocados — can't go in the juicer; they should go in a blender. Like I said earlier, I don't suggest juicing loads of fruit *unless* it's apple or pear. In cases where you have a cold, flu or sinus infection and are looking for a vitamin C boost, I make an exception and juice with a grapefruit and orange. Remember that juices enter the bloodstream quickly, hence you should focus your juices on vegetables, and keep fruit in the blender. Check out all of my recipes for ideas on what to juice and blend.

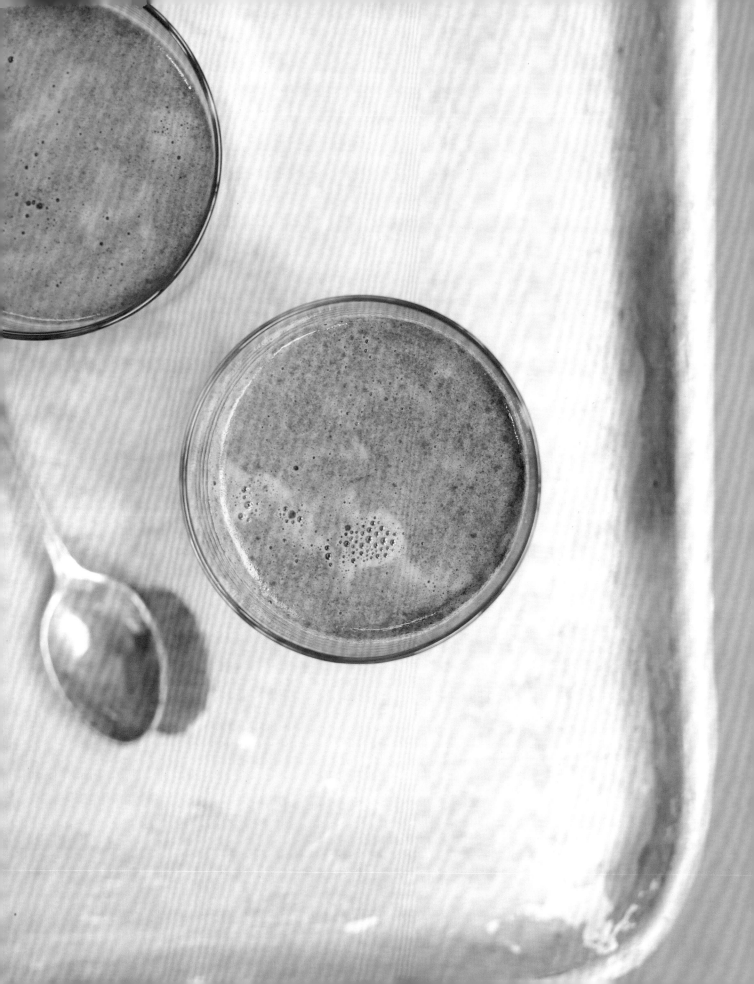

WHEN SHOULD I JUICE OR BLEND?

You can juice any time, but you must consume juice on an empty stomach. Your digestive system will wreak havoc on you if you have a juice less than two hours after eating. Because the vitamins and nutrients enter your bloodstream within twenty minutes, drinking the juice on an empty stomach will allow you to take advantage of the goodness. You should also wait twenty minutes after having your juice before you eat anything.

Blending has a longer absorption process, but it is best to drink your smoothie on an empty stomach. If your smoothie is packed with nutrients and protein you could use this as a breakfast or lunch replacement, but most smoothies are best as a snack. I apply the same rules for juice, and make sure to have the smoothie on an empty stomach and wait to have my next meal. Basically, any time you want a nutritious snack or a quick pick-me-up, grab a juice or smoothie.

Smoothies are more filling than juices and make the perfect snack.

THE BIG PURCHASE

WHAT EQUIPMENT DO I NEED?

Once you have decided between a juicer and blender — or both — take note of the following tips to get you started with the right equipment.

JUICER

There are two main types of juicer and lots of options once you choose which one is right for you:

> » **centrifugal juicer**
>
> » **slow-masticating juicer**

Centrifugal juicer

This is the most popular juicer due to the ease of use, affordability and level of clean-up. This juicer is easy to find in retail shops and online. However, the centrifugal juicer requires that you drink your juice within fifteen minutes of being made. That is because there are live enzymes in the juice and once they are exposed to air they oxidize and their nutritional value decreases.

THE PROS OF A CENTRIFUGAL JUICER

» It is the most affordable juicer.

» It is easy to use.

» It typically takes up less counter space than other juicers.

» Most fruit and vegetables do not need to be pitted, peeled and cut (as long as they fit through the chute).

» It is quicker than using a slow-masticating juicer.

THE CONS OF A CENTRIFUGAL JUICER

» It produces less juice than a slow-masticating juicer, meaning more wastage, so if you are buying a lot of expensive produce you might have your heart broken.

» Fewer nutrients are retained, because fruit and vegetables are shredded with a blade and therefore are exposed to air and oxidize.

» It cannot juice grasses.

» It is not ideal for juicing leafy greens.

» It cannot make nut milks.

» You must drink your juice within fifteen minutes of making it, otherwise you lose the beneficial enzymes.

» It produces foam or froth (some consider this a pro and like this).

» The juice separates.

» The machine is loud.

Slow-masticating juicer

This machine operates by crushing and pressing the fruit and vegetables to squeeze out the juice. It doesn't produce as much heat as a centrifugal juicer, so it keeps the nutrients intact. This juicer is more expensive than a centrifugal juicer, but you will yield a lot more juice and can keep the juice for up to three days in an airtight container in the refrigerator.

THE PROS OF A SLOW-MASTICATING JUICER

» Higher juice yield.

» Higher quality juice because it retains more nutrients.

» It can juice grasses.

» It is optimal for juicing leafy greens.

» Most slow-masticating juicers allow you to make nut milks.

» Juice lasts longer, up to three days after making the juice (in an airtight container).

» It produces minimal foam or froth.

» There is no juice separation.

» The machine is quiet.

THE CONS OF A SLOW-MASTICATING JUICER

» Fruit and vegetables must be cut into 5 cm/2 inch (or smaller) pieces.

» It is more expensive than a centrifugal juicer.

» It requires greater clean-up.

» It is more involved to use than a centrifugal juicer.

Cleaning your juicer

Clean your juicer right after making your juice, each and every time. Don't wait! Clean out the pulp (remember to compost it, give it to your neighbour's chickens or create some new recipes by adding the pulp to your baking), then clean the juicer with water and light soap or as directed in your instruction manual. I am very picky about my equipment, so I use a drying rack and don't allow my juicer or blender near chemicals or the dishwasher.

BLENDER

Blenders vary in cost, size and functionality. There are many blenders that claim to be the best for smoothies, but here are a few things to consider when buying a blender:

» **Power — can the blender handle nut milks and churning vegetables?**

» **Get a glass jug, not plastic.**

» **Tamper — a tamper will allow you to push the ingredients down towards the blade and therefore blend better.**

» **Functionality — what else can the blender do? Make sure it's multi-functional and can help you with cooking and baking as well — unless you just want the blender for smoothies.**

» **Size — is it big enough for what you need but still looks nice on the counter?**

» **Speed — you will need two speeds to blend smoothies.**

» **Cost — a cheap blender is a bad investment; invest in a great-quality blender and know that it could last you a lifetime.**

» **Noise — most will wake up the entire house!**

The most popular blender on the market is the Vitamix, which can do everything a blender should do. Keep in mind, this machine is more costly than most, but for good reason and it will last you a lifetime. There are many options on the market, so do your research and go with what feels best for you.

OTHER EQUIPMENT NEEDED

Here's a shortlist of must-have equipment for juicing and blending. Most of these items may already be in your kitchen, but if not they are worth the investment:

» **Water-filter system or jug — I love alkaline filters (see page 17 to learn more about alkalinity) and can taste the difference, but as long as you are filtering your water you are on the right path (but check out alkaline water filter jugs; I have a feeling you won't be disappointed).**

- » Salad spinner — a must to wash your leafy greens.

- » Colander — for rinsing fruit and vegetables.

- » Vegetable peeler — to make sure you peel away any pesticides.

- » Veggie scrub brush — especially good for scrubbing root vegetables.

- » Lemon/lime squeezer — you can get a fancy hand-held citrus juicer, or my favourite is a wood reamer (they look amazing and store well).

- » Good quality, sharp knife — I also use a sharpener to keep the blade working well.

- » Cutting board — I have a separate board for fruits and vegetables, which has never been touched by animal products.

- » Measuring cup — to measure your liquids.

- » Teaspoons for powders, nut butters and honey

- » Nut milk bag, if you plan to make nut milks — store-bought nut milk (especially in boxes) is filled with preservatives and sugar.

- » Mason jars or tumblers with lids. (You can also get coloured tumblers with lids if you are serving green juices to kids who get squeamish at the colour.)

- » Jugs for nut milk or large batches of juices for serving.

- » Straws for serving.

- » Large bowl — to store fruits and vegetables during preparation.

- » Mild, chemical-free soap — for cleaning the juicer, blender and your equipment.

- » Brush/cleaner for the juicer.

- » Ziplock bags — for freezing fruit, such as peeled bananas for blending.

JOIN A CSA. START A CSA. WHAT'S A CSA?

No farmers' markets in your area? No problem. Investigate a CSA — Community Supported Agriculture Program. When living in New York City, with no farms and no farmers cruising around my neighbourhood, I investigated. I knew there were farmers' markets available on weekends, but that didn't always work for me. I found someone who had started her very own CSA program; she had a van and visited every farmer she knew in upstate New York to pick up loads of fresh, local produce and deliver it right to our office each week. A group of us joined in the fun of never knowing what exciting fruit and vegetables were coming to us each week. We loved it. If you aren't sure where to begin, start with an online search to find farmers in your state. Then call and ask if they know anyone delivering to your area. The farmers I know love this idea and are super helpful. Get the word out, start a CSA!

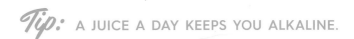

ACIDIC VERSUS ALKALINE

What does it mean to keep the body alkaline, and why? You may have heard of the 'alkaline diet', which states that in order to remain healthy, balanced and free from diseases such as cancer and diabetes, we must eat an 80/20 diet: 80 per cent alkaline foods and 20 per cent acidic foods.

When your body is too acidic you become sick, because disease thrives in an acidic environment. It is easy in today's fast-paced society to slip into poor dietary habits, relying on processed foods, coffee, soft drinks and alcohol; this, combined with stress, can lead to high levels of acidity in your body.

An acidic lifestyle can be the root of constipation, poor digestion, aches, pains, headaches, fatigue, insomnia and a host of serious diseases including the scary Cs: cancer, cardiovascular disease and corpulence. Alkalinity — the antidote to acidity — is achieved by eating more vegetables. The minerals from vegetables, such as calcium, are leached from our bones to alkalise the body, and in addition the body stores fat as a buffer against acidity; therefore a diet high in alkaline foods helps protect you from disease. Start juicing your vegetables every day and you are one step closer to being more alkaline.

Tip: BUY PH SLIPS FROM THE CHEMIST AND TEST YOUR PH LEVELS TO CHECK YOUR ALKALINITY.

How do we eat an 80/20 diet? As well as focusing on alkaline foods and avoiding acidic foods, the answer can be found in juicing — and lots of it! Here are some alkaline foods commonly used in juicing:

- **green vegetables**
- **root vegetables**
- **cucumbers, avocados, tomatoes**
- **lemons, limes, grapefruit**
- **nuts**
- **whole grains.**

Tip: I HAVE BEEN ASKED MANY TIMES HOW LEMON AND LIMES ARE ALKALINE. THEY ARE ACIDIC ON THEIR OWN, BUT ONCE IN THE BODY THEY HAVE AN ALKALIZING EFFECT. ADDING LEMON AND LIME TO YOUR JUICES OR WATER DAILY IS IMPORTANT AND KEEPS YOU ALKALINE.

BUYING YOUR INGREDIENTS

Once you have your equipment, it's time to stock up on those juicy ingredients. Fill your fruit and vegetable trays in the refrigerator so you have enough on hand for a few days, with variety. Grow some herbs in your kitchen or garden. Fill your cupboard with loads of smoothie ingredients.

You can buy produce anywhere, but I strongly suggest you visit a farmers' market or organic grocer. Look to your local health-food stores for smoothie ingredients such as protein powders, nut butters, nuts, cacao and many more of your fun ingredients. Buying in season is key. If you are buying organic, then you are buying seasonal. When you are shopping for your ingredients choose fresh, ripe and organic. I suggest shopping at least twice per week if you are a daily juicer. Leave the brown bananas, mushy avocados and mouldy lemons on the shelves; choose instead ingredients that are in season and ripe.

BUYING ORGANIC: IS IT WORTH IT?

Juicing is truly about putting the best produce in your body. Years ago, eating organic was less of a concern because there weren't as many pesticides in our soil. Now our soil is nutrient depleted, and therefore organic produce is more important and relevant. There is, however, conflicting research on buying organic. Some studies report no difference in nutrition and some report that organic vegetables are higher in vitamins, minerals and phytonutrients. According to naturopath and nutritionist Helen Ridge, we should consume organic produce when possible due to the excess of harmful herbicides and pesticides. Now, that's enough of a reason for me to buy organic. However, we know this is not always possible due to availability and cost. In this case, check out my list overleaf of the 'Dirty Dozen' and 'Clean Fifteen'. The Dirty Dozen has the highest level of pesticides and the Clean Fifteen shows the lowest amount of pesticide residue. Therefore, if you can't always choose organic, use the list.

THE DIRTY DOZEN — BUY ONLY ORGANIC

- » Apples
- » Peaches
- » Nectarines
- » Strawberries
- » Grapes
- » Celery
- » Spinach
- » Capsicum (peppers)
- » Cucumbers
- » Cherry tomatoes
- » Snap peas (mangetout)
- » Potatoes
- » Bonus: Kale

Source: The Environmental Working Group

THE CLEAN FIFTEEN — NO NEED TO BUY ORGANIC

- » Avocados
- » Sweet corn
- » Pineapples
- » Cabbage
- » Peas
- » Onions
- » Asparagus
- » Mangoes
- » Papayas (pawpaw)
- » Kiwi
- » Eggplant (aubergine)
- » Grapefruit
- » Rockmelon (cantaloupe)
- » Cauliflower
- » Sweet potatoes

PREPPING YOUR INGREDIENTS

CLEANING AND PREPPING

If you do nothing else to prep your ingredients, make sure you wash your fruit and vegetables! I used to be the typical lazy juicer who never washed ingredients; I assumed because I was putting organic or locally grown produce in my juicer they would be fine. However, when I thought about all the hands that touched my carrots before I did, I didn't need to remind myself to wash them any more. It's common sense.

The bigger reason to wash your fruit and vegetables, though, is not just germs, but pesticides. We have talked about pesticides and why it is important to buy organic, but I want to share some interesting information on exactly what pesticides do to the body and why it is so important to avoid them. Imagine spraying your garden with insect killer to keep the mosquitos at bay — then eating those leaves you just sprayed. That is what you do when you don't wash your fruit and vegetables. Pesticides can build up in the body, and have been linked to birth defects, hormone disruption, thyroid disease and many other illnesses. Studies that have been conducted on individual produce items say it is safe at a certain level, but as we mix produce the levels of pesticides we put into our body increases, essentially creating a concoction of pesticides. Organic fruit and vegetables are free from these pesticides and therefore don't have the same effect. The bottom line is to buy organic or really wash those ingredients well.

Tip: WASH ALL YOUR FRUIT AND VEGETABLES. ALWAYS.

It is a good idea to wash your fruit and vegetables right away, with the exception of your leafy greens. (The latter tend to wilt, so wash these just before you use them.) Scrub your root vegetables (carrots, sweet potatoes, ginger, beets, kohlrabi and tumeric) with a scrub brush; never use soap unless it is specifically made for cleaning produce. You can easily make your own washing liquid using 1 cup of water with a splash of lemon juice and a splash of white vinegar. I put my liquid wash in a spray bottle and use that to clean my fruit and vegetables. I then rinse them with water in a colander and lay them on a tea towel to dry and then store them.

A little bit of advance preparation can make juicing and blending an easier habit to adopt.

Ideally it would be nice to prepare your ingredients so they are ready to go, but it's best to save the cutting and chopping for when the fruit and vegetables are ready to go into the juicer or blender. Ideally, they will be fresh and therefore will give you a better quality juice or smoothie. However, if the only way you will juice or blend is with a little advance planning, then I say go for it: cut and chop ahead of time. If you use this method, be sure to seal the cut produce in cling wrap and refrigerate.

SOME IDEAS ON HOW TO PREP YOUR PRODUCE

» **Use a salad spinner to wash your leafy greens.**

» **Dry your leafy greens before you refrigerate them.**

» **If juicing: cut or chop your fruit and vegetables so they will easily fit into the juice extractor.**

» **If blending: pit, core and peel your fruit and vegetables.**

FREEZING YOUR INGREDIENTS

Using frozen ingredients is best for blending and making gorgeous, creamy smoothies without adding ice. But there are a few tricks to getting this part of the process right.

I came home from the local farmers' markets and my amazing husband Joe asked if I needed help putting everything away. I jumped with joy, and then I asked him to freeze the bananas and avocados. He took care of it, which meant one less thing for me to do. The next day when I went to make a smoothie I opened the freezer door and found bananas, with the peel on them, and sitting next to them were loose avocados, with the peel and pit still intact! I laughed, and at that moment I knew it was important I included a section in this book on how to freeze your fruit and vegetables. My husband clearly had no idea how to freeze bananas or avocados. Hint: you don't put fruit or vegetables in the freezer unpeeled. First up, here is a list of supplies I use for freezing:

» **reusable freezer bags (BPA-free) or containers**

» **marker pen**

» **chopping board**

» **knife**

» **colander**

» **tea towel**

» **baking sheet and baking paper**

» **ice trays (if you want to prepare leafy greens)**

You have two options when freezing. You can freeze your fruit or vegetables individually — for example, freeze all your strawberries together in one freezer bag and then freeze all your bananas together in another freezer bag. Or, you can freeze everything in bundles — this means you plan your smoothie recipes for the week and put all the ingredients together in one freezer bag. Either option works; it just depends what type of a blender you are. I typically store my ingredients separately and then throw things in and make choices on what to put together as I'm making the smoothie. However, if you like recipes and planning ahead, then the bundles will work well for you. Whatever will get you blending more is the best way to go! Follow these steps to ensure your frozen fruit is ready to go when you are:

1. **Buy ingredients — ripe, in season, organic and local (when possible).**

2. **Wash ingredients.**

3. **Dry ingredients — use a colander and/or tea towel.**

4. **Prep your ingredients — here is a shortlist of ingredients and how to prep:**

    »   **berries (blackberries, blueberries, raspberries) — leave as is**

    »   **strawberries — hull**

    »   **cherries — remove pits and stems**

    »   **stone fruit (peaches, nectarines, plums) — remove pits and cut into pieces**

    »   **oranges — peel and cut in half**

    »   **mangos — peel, remove pits and cut into pieces**

    »   **bananas — make sure they are ripe, peel and cut in half**

    »   **apples, pears — peel, core and cut in half**

    »   **rockmelon (cantaloupe), honeydew — peel, remove seeds and cut into pieces**

    »   **avocado — peel, remove pit and cut in half**

    »   **pineapples — remove spiny top, peel and cut into pieces**

> » leafy greens (spinach or kale) — put in blender, add water and blend — add this to ice-cube trays and freeze (skip the pre-freeze process detailed below).

5.   Pre-freeze prep: Cover a baking tray with a sheet of baking paper. Place all your washed and dried fruit on the tray, with a little space between each piece, and place the tray in the freezer. Allow the fruit to freeze (usually at least six hours), then, using a spatula, pull the fruit off the baking tray, place in bags, label and place the bags in the freezer. If you decide to skip this step, make sure your fruit is dry before putting it into bags.

6.   Label your freezer bags with the ingredient and date — add ingredients to bags (either in smoothie bundles or by fruit).

7.   Freeze and use within two months.

Tip: THE BASIC RULES TO FREEZING YOUR FRUIT AND VEGETABLES ARE: BUY, WASH, DRY, PREP, LABEL AND FREEZE. *VOILÀ!* ... DELICIOUS SMOOTHIES!

STORING YOUR INGREDIENTS

Here are some suggestions on how to store your fruit and vegetables, depending on climate. (If you are in a hot or humid climate, this may not work for you — I learned this the hard way after moving from New York to Sydney and discovering fruit flies.)

> » **Herbs do really well on the counter top and look like a nice decoration — I put them in a small vase or glass of water.**

> » **Leafy greens do best in the vegetable drawer in your refrigerator, unwashed.**

> » **Carrots and beets are best in the refrigerator, scrubbed with a scrub brush.**

- » **I leave all stone fruit (peaches, nectarines, plums), apples, pears, pineapple, lemons, limes, bananas and avocado in a decorative bowl on my counter (or a cool area in warmer months), or I freeze some of these items for smoothies.**

- » **I store berries (raspberries, blueberries, strawberries, blackberries) in the freezer (see the section on how to freeze fruit and vegetables).**

STORING YOUR JUICE

Your juices are alive and full of vitamins, minerals and enzymes. They don't have any added preservatives and therefore don't have a shelf life. For the freshest juice I recommend always drinking your juice right away. (As I have noted, if you are using a centrifugal juicer you must drink your juice within fifteen minutes, and within three days or 72 hours if using a slow-masticating juicer.) If you don't drink your juice right away then it needs to be refrigerated in an airtight container.

You should also drink your smoothies right away, to obtain the benefits of the nutrients. You can keep the smoothies for 24 to 72 hours in an airtight container in the refrigerator.

SIMPLE RECIPE MIXERS

While recipes are fun, sometimes it's easier to throw your own ingredients together based on what you have in your kitchen. Here are two simple recipes that can help you create your own juicy and smoothie goodness. Have fun with it and feel free to experiment with different ingredients!

SIMPLE GREEN JUICE — YOUR WAY

Let's keep it green, healthy and full of vitamins and minerals. Consume your daily vegetables with one green delicious juice!

For this recipe you will need: juicer, citrus reamer, knife, cutting board, glass to drink. Choose **one** from each of the following.

CHOOSE 1 LEAFY GREEN
- » 1 large handful kale leaves
- » 1 large handful spinach
- » 1 large handful lettuce (cos or romaine)
- » 2 large handfuls rocket (arugula)
- » 1 large handful silverbeet

THEN 1 GREEN HERB
- » 1 handful coriander (cilantro)
- » 1 handful mint
- » 1 handful parsley
- » 1 handful basil

1 BASE
- » 1 cucumber
- » 4 stalks celery

1 FRUIT FOR SWEETNESS
- » 1 pear
- » 1 apple

AND ADD 1
- » ½ lemon, keep peel on for squeezing
- » 1 large knob ginger

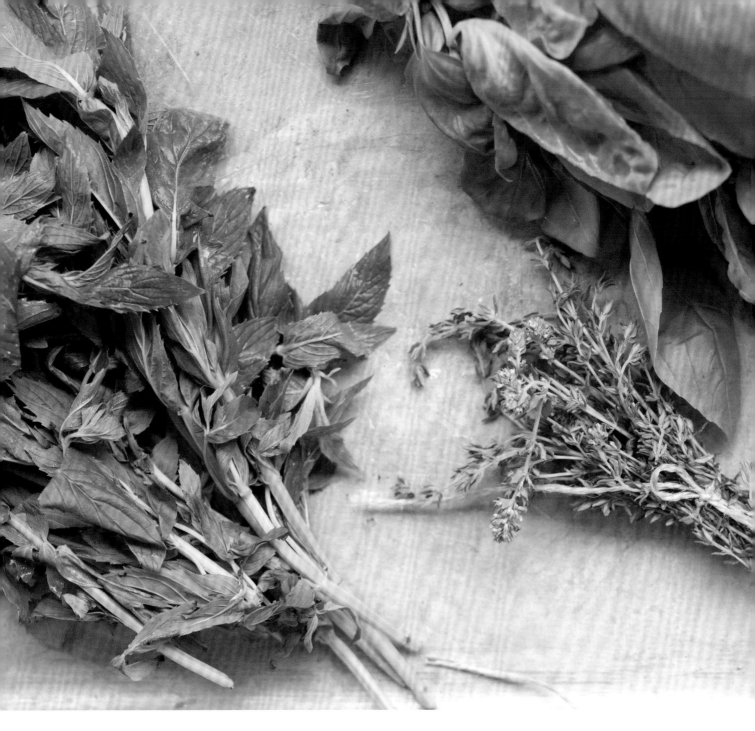

Follow these prep directions for the ingredients you selected. Cut the cucumber in half. Cut the celery stalks to fit into the juicer. Cut the apple or pear to fit into the juicer.

Wash vegetables. Place your leafy greens, herbs, cucumber or celery, apple or pear and ginger (if using) into the juicer and run the machine. Pour the Simple Green Juice into your glass. Using your citrus reamer, squeeze the lemon into your juice and enjoy the perfect, yummy green juice.

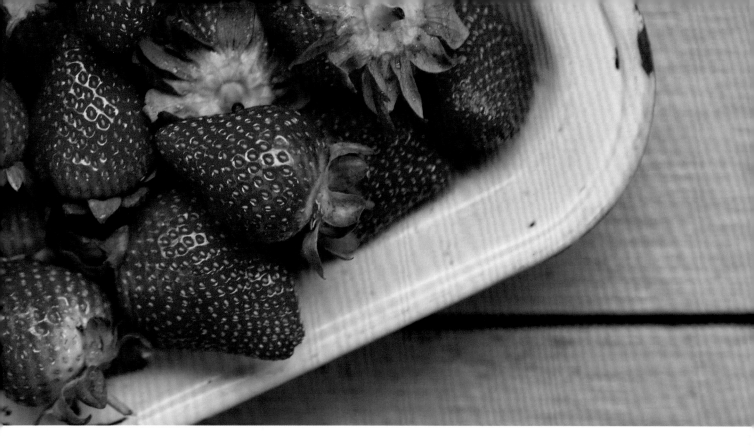

SIMPLE SMOOTHIE — YOUR WAY

Let's keep it real. No dairy. No added sugar. When we talk smoothies, we are talking health, not sugar-filled dairy treats. Add what you please, but keep it healthy!

For this recipe you will need: blender, measuring cup, knife, cutting board, teaspoon, tablespoon, mason jar or glass to drink, straw.

Choose one from each of the following.

LIQUID

»   **1 cup almond milk***

»   **1 cup cashew milk***

»   **1 cup coconut water**

»   **1 cup filtered water**

Use my homemade recipe (see pages 58 and 59) for the best, nutrition- and health-packed nut milk

ADD

»   **1 banana, peeled and frozen**

BERRY	» 1 cup blueberries, frozen
	» 1 cup strawberries, stemmed and frozen
	» 1 cup raspberries, frozen
VEGETABLE	(optional, but an added health bonus)
	» 1 small handful leafy greens: kale, spinach, lettuce or rocket (arugula)
POWDER	(optional, but great for added protein):
	» 1 tablespoon protein powder, such as pea, hemp or rice (I stay away from whey protein, which is dairy, and use something that is vegan and easily digested)
ONE OR TWO SUPERFOODS	» 1 tablespoon cacao powder
	» 1 handful cacao nibs
	» 1 teaspoon maca powder (Peruvian ginseng)
	» 1 teaspoon flax seeds
	» 1 teaspoon chia seeds
FOR ADDED LOVE, CHOOSE ONE	» 1 tablespoon nut butter (ABC, almond or cashew)
	» 1 medjool date

Follow the prep directions for the ingredients you selected. For most of the fruit I use in smoothies, I prepare and freeze them first (check out my section on prepping your ingredients, page 20). Prepping and freezing your fruit means no adding ice to your smoothies, which makes your smoothies thicker and more delicious.

Prepare all of your ingredients. Wash your leafy green vegetables (if adding). Add your liquid, banana, berries, greens, powder, superfoods and nut butter or date to the blender and run the machine. Using the tamper, move your ingredients around for best consistency. Pour the Simple Smoothie into your glass or jar. Top it with your straw and enjoy this perfect, yummy simple fruit and protein smoothie!

SOME FINAL TIPS

» For a balance of vitamins and minerals, don't eat the same greens every day.

» Shop at least twice a week if you are a daily juicer.

» Leave the brown bananas, mushy avocados and mouldy lemons on the shelves. Choose ingredients that are in season and ripe.

» To keep your body alkaline, stick to three vegetables and one fruit in your juices. There are loads of recipes to choose from, but when in doubt use my simple green easy customized recipe (see page 26).

» Choose a juice or smoothie over a shot of espresso when you need your afternoon energizer.

» Don't trash your pulp! Learn to bake with it. Compost it and grow a gorgeous garden. Feed it to the chickens!

» Always use glass or BPA-free bottles for your juices and smoothies.

» Buy a water filter, for your daily water intake and smoothies.

» Freeze your fruit for smoothies. Don't add ice!

» Juice every single day.

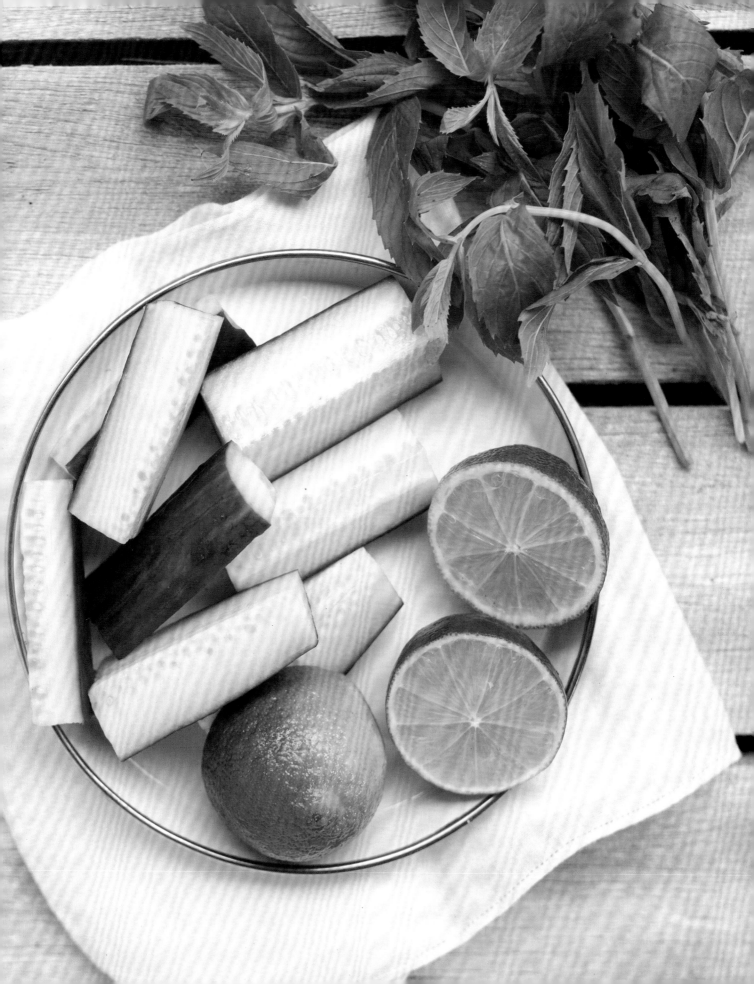

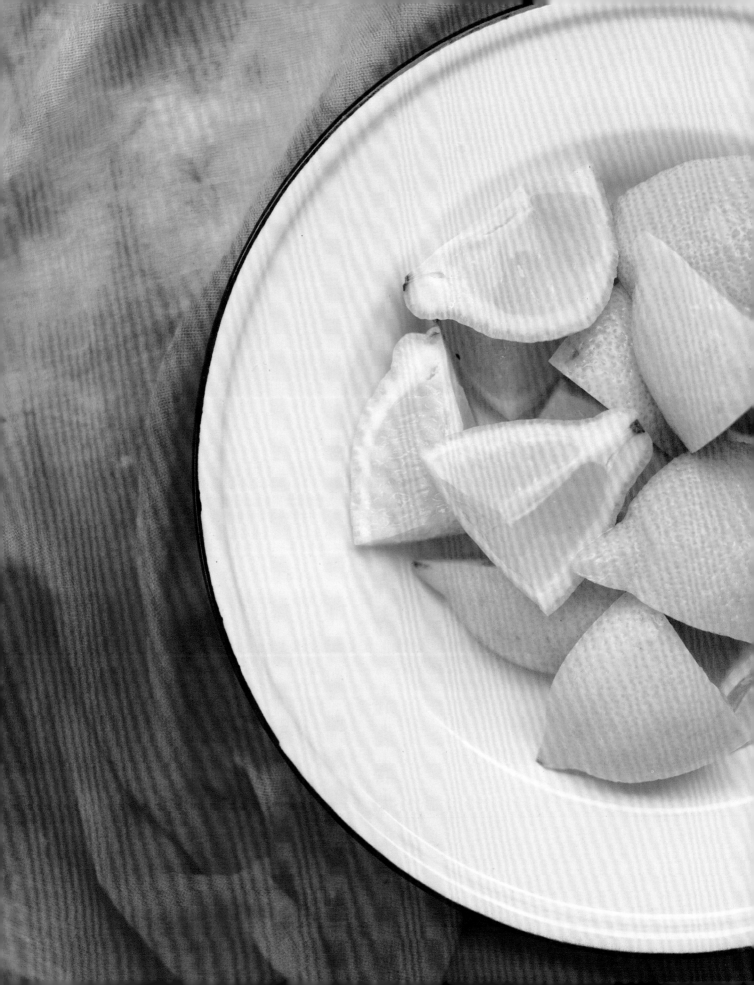

CHAPTER 2

MORNING RITUAL

It's important you create a morning ritual that resonates with you, because that way you'll be able to make it part of your routine for life. Here are some techniques I incorporate into my life — some or all of these might work for you:

» Wake early and naturally. Forget the alarm. I leave my window blinds open so I can rise with the sun; it's a wonderful, peaceful way to wake up.

» Breathing and mantras. Before I get out of bed I start with deep, slow breathing. I also use a mantra — a word or phrase repeated to still the mind — that helps me focus on the new day. A beautiful mantra could be to help you restore your health, such as, '*I treat my body with love and heal it with green juice*'. The beauty of a mantra is that it can be whatever you want it to be.

» Hot water and lemon. The first thing I put in my body each day is a glass of boiled water, cooled to room temperature, with a squeeze of lemon. Remember that lemon is alkalizing and high in vitamin C, which helps to begin the fat-burning process.

» Morning stretch. All the green juice in the world wouldn't be enough if I didn't incorporate yoga into my daily life. There are many poses and sequences you can do to start your day. Begin with simple poses for your morning stretch. If you are new to stretching, there are plenty of great websites and phone apps out there to help you along.

A good start to the morning is a great start to the day!

» Set intentions. They say without having an intention there is no intention. Therefore, each morning I calmly think about what I intend for the day, and I make a list of things I want to accomplish. If I focus the morning around being good to myself, the rest of the day then generally comes with grace and ease.

» Gratitude journal. It's so important to think about those in your life whom you love and how you are grateful to them for the goodness they have brought you. You can do this verbally, but I find keeping a journal is helpful and a way to reflect on my feelings.

» Aloe Vera juice. I love this easy morning cleanse. A shot of aloe vera is full of vitamins and minerals, high in essential fatty acids, helps with digestion, alkalizes the body, helps with weight loss and boosts your immune system.

» Alkaline water. Alkaline water is pure and tastes beautiful. But, as long as you filter your water and keep it clean you are on the right track. I suggest drinking 2 litres/4 pints or eight glasses of water per day and twelve glasses with a deep cleanse or detox.

» Go green — green juice! Adding chlorophyll to your life will keep you grounded, calm and anxiety free. Dark leafy greens are alkalizing and create balance to start the day off right.

» I focus the morning around being good to myself, calmly making lists and thoughts for what I want to accomplish that day; the rest of the day then generally comes with grace and ease.

OIL PULLING AND TONGUE SCRAPING

Oil pulling is a powerful healing treatment that changed my life, my teeth and my morning.

Simple Oil Pulling

1. Place 1 teaspoon of organic cold-pressed coconut oil in your mouth and swish around for twenty minutes, making sure not to swallow (you may gag and need to spit out the oil in less time when you are starting out).

2. After twenty minutes, spit the oil into the rubbish or toilet bowl (do not spit in the sink, because you will clog the drain).

3. Rinse your mouth with water.

4. Tongue scrape (see below).

5. Brush your teeth using toothpaste.

Tongue scraping helps remove toxins. After oil pulling or when you wake up in the morning, use a copper or aluminium tongue scraper to scrape your tongue for five scrapes, cleaning it with water after each scrape.

THE BENEFITS OF FRUIT AND VEGETABLES IN THE MORNING

» Beets contain nitrate, which gives us more stamina, lowers blood pressure and fights inflammation.

» Berries start the day off right by increasing our memory and learning potential. Adding berries to our smoothies or juices is a great benefit for both adults and children.

» Spinach provides balance and co-ordination, helping to set us up for a productive day.

» Pineapple contains the enzyme bromelain, which is said to reduce inflammation, joint pain and protects us from tumour growth. Bromelain is also said to heal wounds, support digestion and prevent constipation as well as be a source of vitamin C, which battles free radicals known to cause cancer.

» Grapefruit is a hydrating fruit, with over 90 per cent water. Incorporating a grapefruit into your daily regime will give you over 50 per cent of your daily vitamin C needs, supporting your immune system and helping fight off colds and flu. This is also an alkaline fruit once digested and therefore has a positive effect on the body and digestive system.

» Chlorophyll has so many amazing benefits. First, it regenerates, cleanses and re-boots the body. It increases blood cells, which improves oxygen absorption. Chlorophyll curbs cravings and therefore helps with weight loss, encourages healing and has amazing potential to fight cancer. They say the darker the green vegetable the higher in chlorophyll it is, so go for a rich green juice or smoothie in the morning.

Tip: IN THE MORNING LIQUIDS ARE EASIEST ON THE DIGESTIVE SYSTEM. SOLID FOODS ARE TOUGH, SO START THE DAY OFF RIGHT WITH A JUICE OR SMOOTHIE!

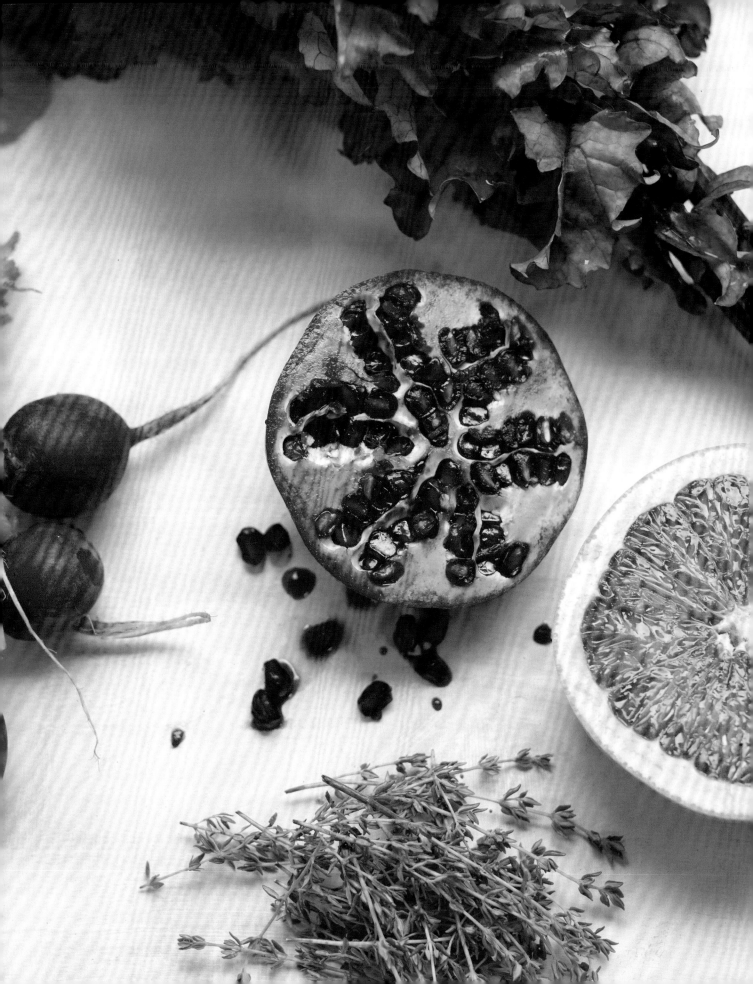

JUICY RECIPES

Tip: JUICES ARE BEST CONSUMED IMMEDIATELY, BUT IF YOU HAVE A SLOW-MASTICATING JUICER YOU CAN STORE YOUR JUICE FOR UP TO THREE DAYS IN AN AIRTIGHT CONTAINER IN THE REFRIGERATOR.

KALE APPLE JUICE

1	green apple
1	handful kale
2	stalks celery
½	cucumber
1	knob ginger

Cut the apple to fit into the juicer. Feed all the ingredients through the juicer. Pour into a glass and serve immediately. Enjoy!

FULL OF GREENS JUICE

1	handful spinach
½	cucumber
1	handful cos (romaine) lettuce
3	stalks celery
1	sprig parsley
1	lemon

Feed the spinach, cucumber, lettuce, celery and parsley through the juicer. Pour into a glass. Using your citrus reamer, squeeze the lemon directly into your juice. Serve immediately. Enjoy!

TUSCAN GREEN JUICE

1	handful Tuscan kale
¼	cucumber
3	broccoli florets
1	handful spinach
2	stalks celery
1	knob ginger
½	lemon

Feed the kale, cucumber, broccoli, spinach, celery and ginger through the juicer. Pour into a glass. Using your citrus reamer, squeeze the lemon directly into your juice. Serve immediately. Enjoy!

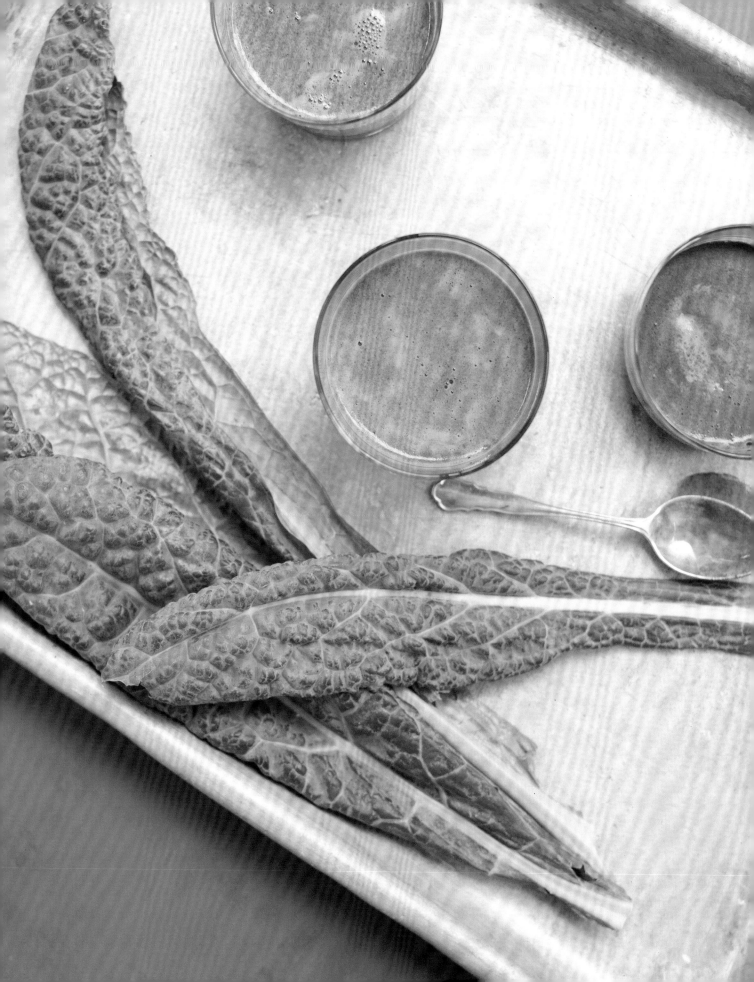

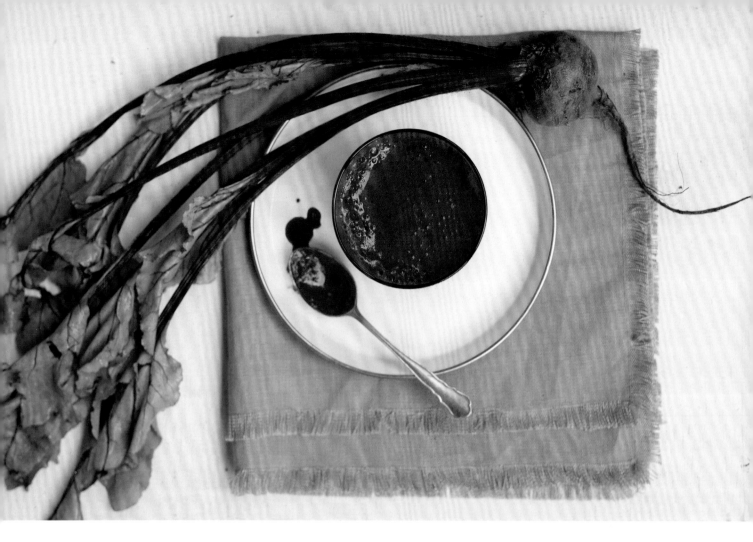

APPLE BEET JUICE

1 beet
1 apple
1 handful mint

Cut the beet and apple to fit into the juicer. Feed the beet, mint and apple through the juicer. Pour into a glass and serve immediately. Enjoy!

GREEN VEGETABLE JUICE

5 broccoli florets
1 cucumber
1 handful parsley
1 lemon

Feed the broccoli, cucumber and parsley through the juicer. Pour into a glass. Using your citrus reamer, squeeze the lemon directly into your juice. Serve immediately. Enjoy!

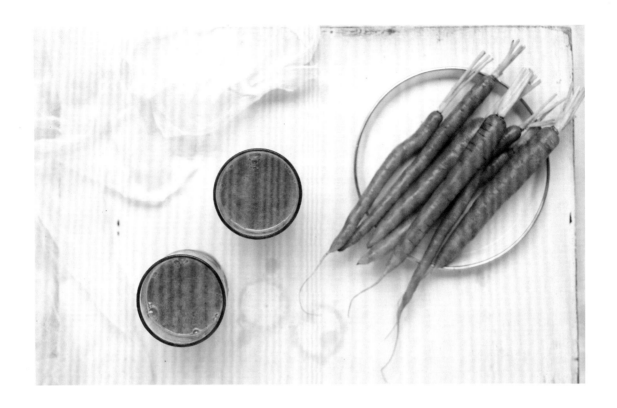

GRAPEFRUIT CARROT JUICE

1 grapefruit
3 carrots
1 knob ginger

Cut the grapefruit in half, then peel and remove the pith, and cut the grapefruit to fit into the juicer. Cut the tips off the carrots. Feed the grapefruit, carrots and ginger through the juicer. Pour into a glass and serve immediately. Enjoy!

VITALITY JUICE

1 tomato
3 carrots
5 stalks celery
1 lemon

Cut the tomato in half to fit into the juicer. Cut the tips off the carrots. Feed the tomato, carrots and celery through the juicer. Pour into a glass. Using your citrus reamer, squeeze the lemon directly into your juice. Serve immediately. Enjoy!

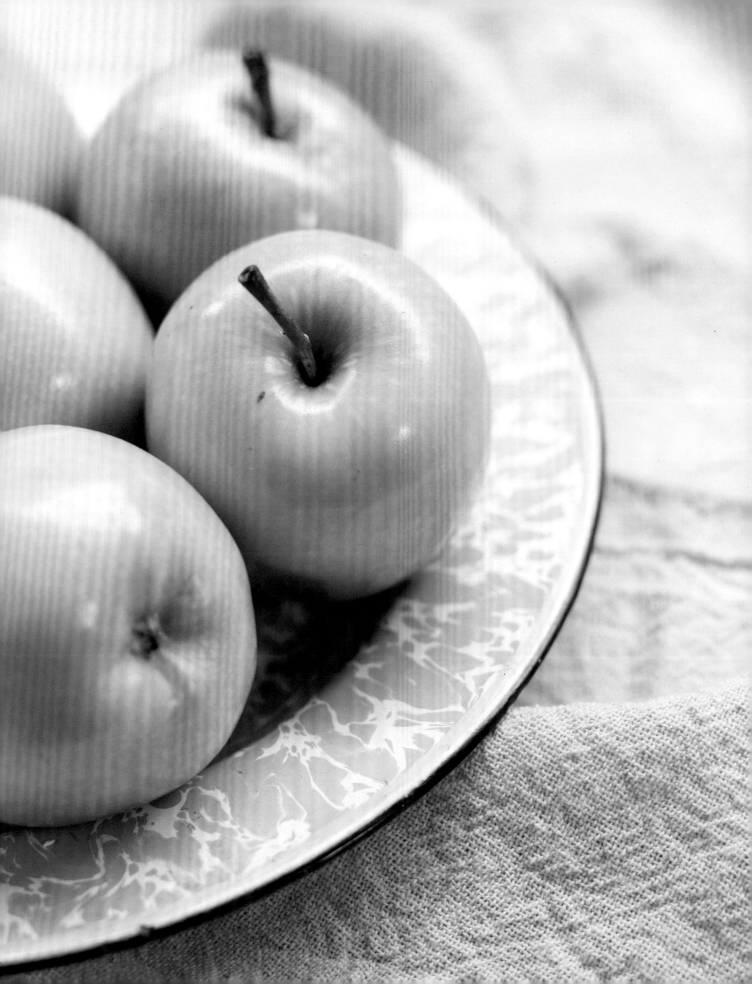

SWEET MORNING GREEN JUICE

½ apple
¼ honeydew melon
1 handful spinach
1 cucumber
1 sprig parsley
2 stalks celery
1 knob ginger

Cut the apple to fit into the juicer. Peel the honeydew melon and cut to fit into the juicer. Feed all the ingredients through the juicer. Pour into a glass and serve immediately. Enjoy!

CARROT APPLE JUICE

5 carrots
2 apples

Cut the tips off the carrots. Cut the apples to fit into the juicer. Feed the carrots and apples through the juicer. Pour into a glass and serve immediately. Enjoy!

PINEAPPLE SPICE JUICE

¼ pineapple
1 handful coriander (cilantro)
½ cucumber
1 small jalapeño

Peel the pineapple and cut to fit into the juicer. Feed all the ingredients through the juicer. Pour into a glass and serve immediately. Enjoy!

SIMPLE SPINACH JUICE

1 handful spinach
1 cucumber
3-4 stalks celery

Feed all the ingredients through the juicer. Pour into a glass and serve immediately. Enjoy!

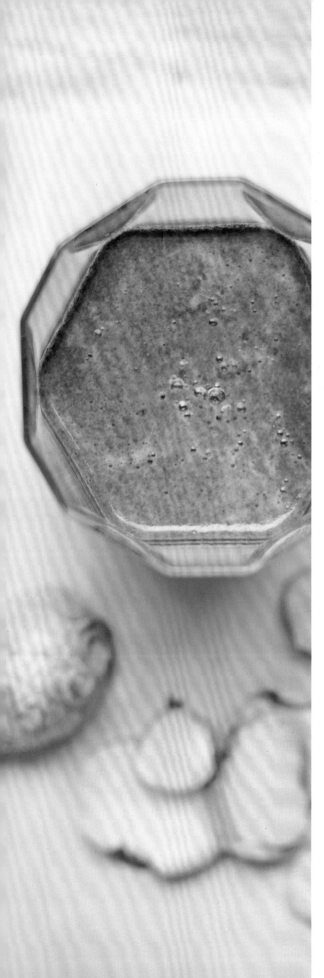

MIXED VEGETABLE JUICE

1 beet
½ apple
1 handful spinach
1 handful kale
1 stalk celery
2 carrots
½ lemon

Cut the beet and apple to fit into the juicer. Feed the beet, apple, spinach, kale, celery and carrots through the juicer. Pour into a glass. Using your citrus reamer, squeeze the lemon directly into your juice. Serve immediately. Enjoy!

MORNING RITUAL GREEN JUICE

½ grapefruit
1 pear
1 handful kale
2 stalks celery
1 cucumber
1 knob ginger

Cut the grapefruit in half, then peel and remove the pith. Cut the grapefruit and pear to fit into the juicer. Feed all the ingredients through the juicer. Pour into a glass and serve immediately. Enjoy!

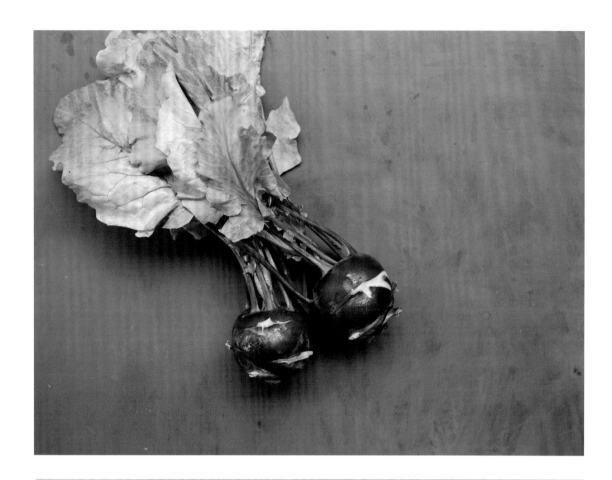

SWEET BEET JUICE

2   beets and beet greens
½   apple
3   carrots

Cut the beets and apple to fit into the juicer. Cut the tips off the carrots. Feed all the ingredients through the juicer. Pour into a glass and serve immediately. Enjoy! .

KOHLRABI JUICE

1   whole kohlrabi
5   carrots

Cut the kohlrabi to fit into the juicer. Cut the tips off the carrots. Feed all the ingredients through the juicer. Pour into a glass and serve immediately. Enjoy!

SOUR GRAPEFRUIT JUICE

1	grapefruit
1	lemon
1	knob ginger

Cut the grapefruit in half, then peel and remove the pith. Peel the lemon and remove the pith. Cut the grapefruit and lemon to fit into the juicer. Feed all the ingredients though the juicer. Pour into a glass and serve immediately. Enjoy!

GINGER SHOT

1	lemon
2	knobs ginger
1	pinch cayenne pepper

Peel the lemon and remove the pith, then cut to fit into the juicer. Feed the lemon and ginger though the juicer. Pour into a glass. Sprinkle the cayenne over the finished juice. Serve immediately. Enjoy!

GRAPEFRUIT THYME JUICE

2	grapefruits
1	sprig thyme

Cut the grapefruits in half, then peel and remove the pith, and cut the grapefruits to fit into the juicer. Feed the grapefruit through the juicer. Pour into a glass. Add the thyme and serve immediately. Enjoy!

COCONUT SWEET KALE SMOOTHIE

½	cup mango, fresh or preferably frozen
1	handful kale
½	cup chopped pineapple, rind removed, fresh or preferably frozen
1	cup coconut water

Peel the mango. Cut the kale and mango into pieces. Add all the ingredients to the blender. Blend and enjoy!

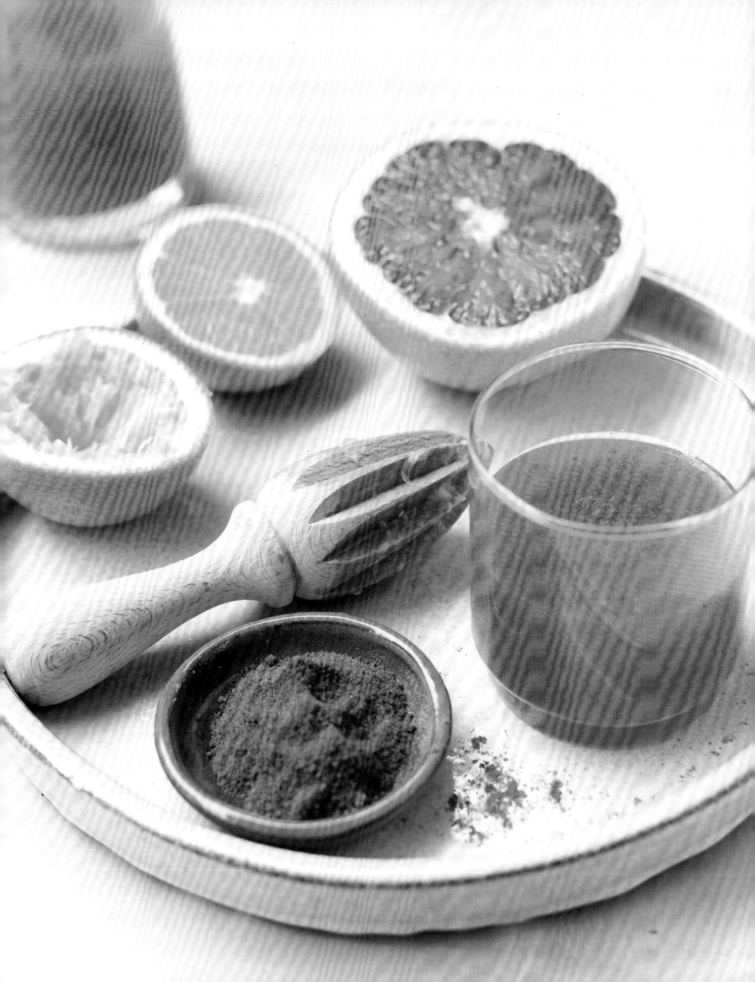

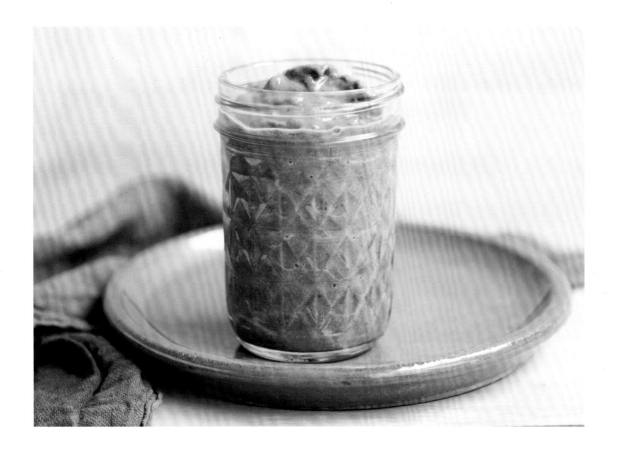

SWEET COCONUT SMOOTHIE

2 oranges
1 cup strawberries, fresh or preferably frozen
1 cup coconut water
1 cup blueberries, fresh or preferably frozen

Peel the oranges and cut into pieces. Hull the strawberries. Add all the ingredients to a blender. Blend and enjoy!

KALE PINEAPPLE SMOOTHIE

½ pineapple, fresh or preferably frozen
1 handful kale
1 cup almond milk (see homemade almond milk recipe, page 58)

Peel the pineapple and cut into pieces. Cut the kale into pieces. Add all the ingredients to a blender. Blend and enjoy!

BERRY APPLE SMOOTHIE

1 banana, fresh or preferably
frozen

1 apple

1 knob ginger

1 cup almond milk
(see homemade almond milk
recipe, page 58)

1 cup berries (blackberries,
blueberries and/or
raspberries), fresh or
preferably frozen

Peel the banana and cut in half. Cut
the apple into pieces. Peel the ginger.
Add all the ingredients to a blender.
Blend and enjoy!

BLUEBERRY COCONUT SMOOTHIE

1 banana, fresh
or preferably frozen

½ cup coconut water

½ cup coconut milk (see
homemade recipe, page 60)

1 cup blueberries, fresh
or preferably frozen

1 teaspoon raw honey

Peel the banana and cut in half. Add
all the ingredients to a blender. Blend
and enjoy!

ACAI SMOOTHIE IN A BOWL

1 banana, fresh

1 tablespoon acai berry
powder

1 cup berries (blackberries,
blueberries and/or
raspberries), fresh or
preferably frozen

1 cup toasted muesli
(or granola)

1 handful shredded coconut

Peel the banana and slice. Add the
acai and berries to a blender. Blend
and add the acai mix to a bowl of
toasted muesli. Top with the banana
and coconut. Enjoy!

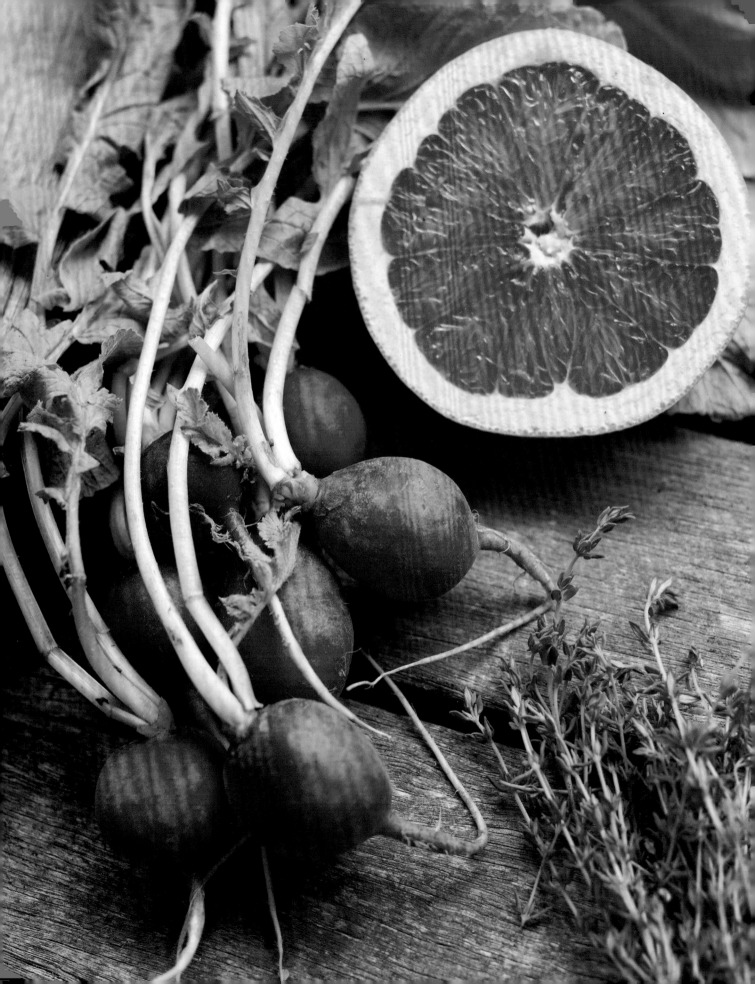

CHAPTER 3

AFTERNOON ENERGIZER

Do you ever experience the afternoon slump? Grab a coffee to stay awake? Sit dreaming of a hammock on the beach with a good book and someone bringing you a rum punch ... I mean, a green juice? By now you know that a coffee or cocktail isn't likely to give you that sparkling energy you were hoping for. Instead of going for something that's harmful to your beautiful body, grab coconut water and one of my healthy juices or smoothies. These will give you energy *the natural way.*

First, other than juices and smoothies, here are a few ways to boost your energy this afternoon:

» **Get up. Stand up and walk around in nature. I suggest an afternoon yoga class, a walk through the park or at the very least a walk around your office or house. Take your meeting on the road; walk with your colleague and get inspired in nature.**

» Stretch. The best afternoon addition to your juice or smoothie is to stretch and wake up your body. When I was managing human resources I incorporated a yoga class into the workplace. We made sure to do the class in a quiet space, pumping up our energy the natural way. So, partner with your local yoga guru and ask them to come in and support this amazing concept of bringing yoga and stretching to you while at work. If you're at home, try a local yoga class or a simple walk in nature.

» Listen to music. Update your playlist and listen to some of your favourite tunes to wake you up and give you a natural high!

» Get cold. Dive into a pool or take a trip to the restroom and splash some cold water on your face. It's my favourite time of day to wash my face and freshen up.

» Skip the fake energy and sugar. Look for natural energy boosters, such as leafy greens or cacao, to add to your smoothies.

HEALTHY ADDITIVES

Let's look inside a few of the powerful ingredients that can help pump you up with energy in the afternoon — or any time. I'm a firm believer that natural energy is sustainable whereas caffeine, sugar, artificial sweeteners (which are my absolute no-no) and store-bought energy drinks give you a false sense of energy and actually kill your mood. These quick pick-me-up boosters mask your real energy and do nothing for your creative juices. In fact, they will leave you with less energy. Instead, give one of these energy boosters a try:

» Coconut oil supports your immune system, which fights off bad bacteria in your gut. Additionally, coconut oil is absorbed into your system immediately, giving you an energy boost.

» Coconut water is nature's natural sports energy drink. Coconut water is hydrating, full of potassium and replaces water and salt, which is ideal after fluid loss, so it's an ideal post-exercise drink.

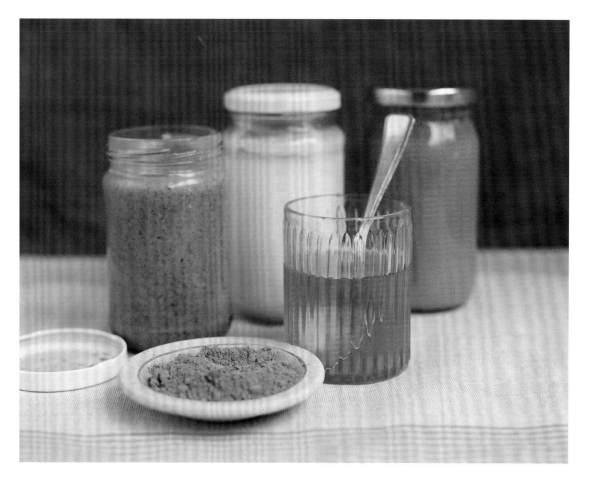

» Coconut milk is simply coconut meat and water — but only if you make it yourself. If you choose the box or canned version, you will also be taking in additives and preservatives that are necessary to give it a long shelf life, but aren't the best for you. Therefore, make your own coconut milk with no additives and get hydrated, fight off harmful bacteria and get fit!

» Nuts and nut milk (almond, Brazil, cashew, walnut and many more) are full of power and protein. They give us an energy boost, fight inflammation and are easily digestible.

FRUIT AND VEGETABLES

» Goji berries are loaded with vitamins C and E; amazing antioxidants that support our immune system, help to fight disease and work to increase energy.

» Bananas are the best natural source of potassium, as well as vitamins B6 and C and fibre. Known as a disease fighter, bananas are an antioxidant that supports our immune system and wakes us up.

» Berries (blackberries, blueberries, raspberries, strawberries and acai berries) are full of antioxidants that keep our brain working. They are a powerhouse for burning fat, therefore exercise and drink your berries!

» Leafy greens are an immune supporter, as well as being packed with vitamins — including A, B, C and K — and minerals that give an all-natural pick-me-up all day long.

POWDERS

» Protein powders (hemp, pea, rice) provide our body with healing and support our immune system, as well as helping to satisfy cravings.

» Maca powder (Peruvian ginseng) is a superfood full of vitamins, such as the B-group and C, iron and calcium. Maca is known to increase energy, and improve libido and fertility.

» Blue-green algae can provide us with vitamin B12, which helps fight fatigue and low energy.

» Chlorella is a super algae and a fantastic source of iron, and comes in the form of a beautiful rich green powder.

» Raw cacao is a superfood that will provide you with antioxidants, protein, iron and fibre. The powder form is my favourite and typically turns your smoothie a deep brown colour that will help you believe you are drinking chocolate.

SWEETENERS

» Coconut nectar, honey and dates are great natural sweeteners. Avoid others — you are sweet enough without them!

JUICY RECIPES

Instead of an afternoon coffee, try the following delicious recipes for a pick-me-up. Some are filled with chlorophyll, which will give you lasting energy.

LOVE YOUR GREENS JUICE

½ lemon
1 handful kale
1 handful spinach
1 small cucumber
4 stalks celery
1 handful parsley
1 knob ginger

Remove the peel and pith of the lemon and cut to fit into the juicer. Feed all the ingredients through the juicer. Pour into a glass and serve immediately. Enjoy!

GREEN ENERGIZER JUICE

1 apple
1 handful spinach
½ large cucumber
3 stalks kale
1 lemon

Cut the apple to fit into the juicer. Feed the apple, spinach, cucumber and kale through the juicer. Pour into a glass. Using your citrus reamer, squeeze the lemon directly into your juice. Serve immediately. Enjoy!

GREEN APPLE JUICE

1 apple, green or gala
1 handful kale
1 handful spinach
1 knob ginger
1 lemon

Cut the apple to fit into the juicer. Feed the apple, kale, spinach and ginger through the juicer. Pour into a glass. Using your citrus reamer, squeeze the citrus directly into your juice. Serve immediately. Enjoy!

SWEET CARROT JUICE

1	beet
½	sweet potato
1	apple
4	carrots
2	stalks celery

Cut the beet, sweet potato and apple to fit into the juicer. Feed all the ingredients through the juicer. Pour into a glass and serve immediately. Enjoy!

SWEET KALE JUICE

¼	pineapple
1	handful kale
1	small cucumber
1	handful chard
1	handful parsley
1	knob ginger

Peel the pineapple and cut to fit into the juicer. Feed all the ingredients through the juicer. Pour into a glass and serve immediately. Enjoy!

BASIL TURMERIC ENERGIZER JUICE

1	apple
1	cucumber
1	handful kale
1	handful basil
1	slice turmeric
1	knob ginger

Cut the apple to fit into the juicer. Feed the ingredients through the juicer. Pour into a glass and serve immediately. Enjoy!

Tip: IF YOU CAN'T FIND FRESH TURMERIC, USE 1 TEASPOON OF GROUND TURMERIC POWDER. ADD THIS TO YOUR GLASS AFTER YOU HAVE POURED THE JUICE. STIR AND ENJOY!

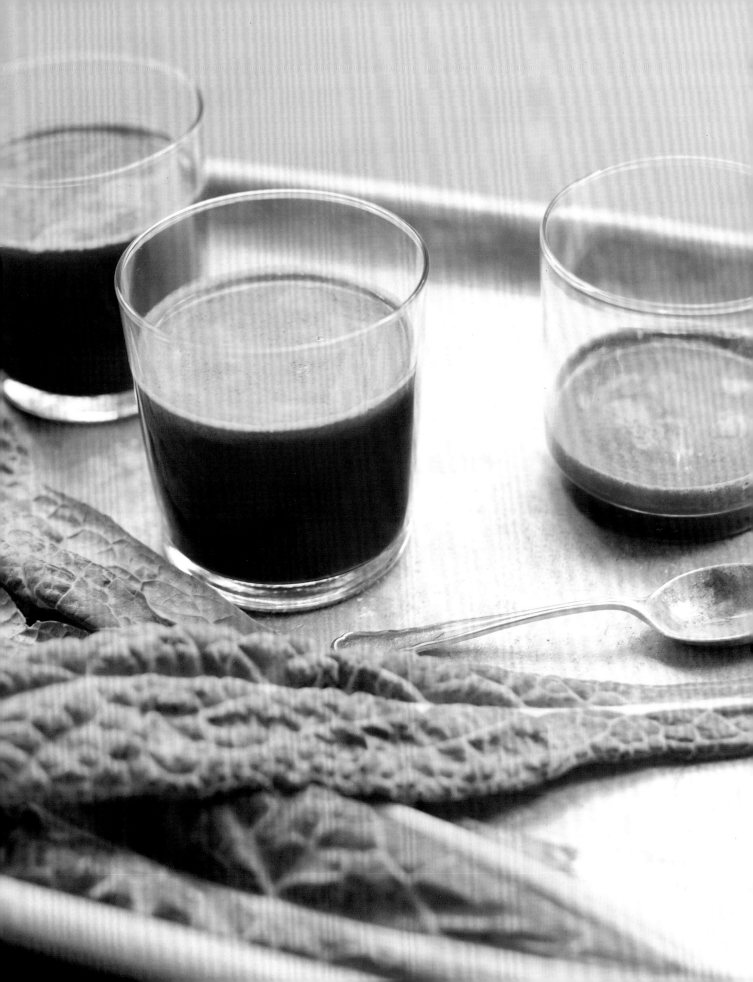

ALMOND MILK — UNSWEETENED

pinch of sea salt
1 cup almonds
4 cups filtered water, plus extra for soaking
nut milk bag

In a glass bowl, cover the almonds with filtered water, add the sea salt and soak overnight, or for a minimum of 8 hours. Discard the soaking liquid and rinse the almonds in water. Add the almonds and 4 cups of filtered water to the blender. Blend until smooth (1–2 minutes). Strain the almonds through the nut milk bag and then transfer to an airtight container (I suggest mason jars). Refrigerate and use within three days. Shake well before using.

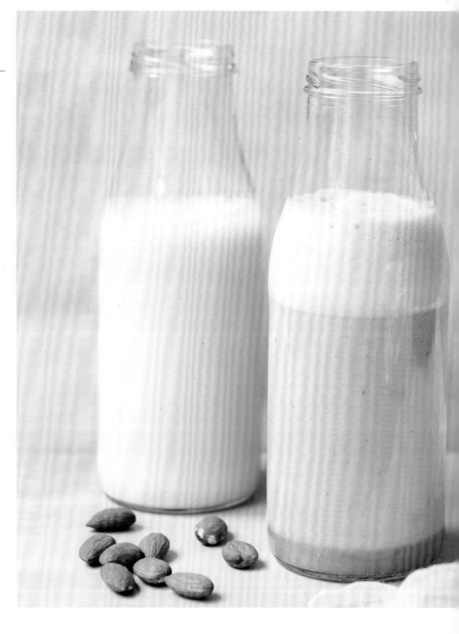

Tip: IF YOU ARE USING A VITAMIX, YOU MAY NOT NEED TO USE A NUT MILK BAG.

Tip: I DON'T RECOMMEND USING CHEESECLOTH; IF YOU DO CHOOSE THIS METHOD, BE SURE TO USE DOUBLE CHEESECLOTH, AND NOTICE THAT THE MILK WILL NOT HAVE THE SAME SMOOTH CONSISTENCY.

NUT MILK — UNSWEETENED

1–2 cups nuts (Brazil, cashew, hazelnut, macadamia or walnut)

4 cups filtered water, plus extra for soaking

nut milk bag

Nut soaking suggestions:
Brazil: minimum 2 hours
Cashew: minimum 2 hours
Hazelnut: minimum 8 hours
Macadamia: minimum 2 hours
Walnut: minimum 4 hours
Note: Do not soak nuts longer than overnight.

In a glass bowl, cover the nuts with filtered water and soak as suggested. Discard the soaking liquid and rinse the nuts in water. Add the nuts and 4 cups of filtered water to the blender. Blend until smooth (1–2 minutes). Strain the nuts through the nut milk bag and then transfer to an airtight container (I suggest mason jars). Refrigerate and use within three days. Shake well before using.

Tip: I MAKE ALL MY NUT MILKS UNSWEETENED BECAUSE I USE THEM FOR SMOOTHIES AND THEY ARE OFTEN SWEET ENOUGH WITH THE BANANA OR ADDED FRUIT.

Tip: SOAKING YOUR NUTS INCREASES THE VITAMIN AVAILABILITY IN THE NUTS AND PROMOTES HEALTHY DIGESTION, AS WELL AS REMOVING THE ANTI-NUTRIENTS AND ENZYME INHIBITORS.

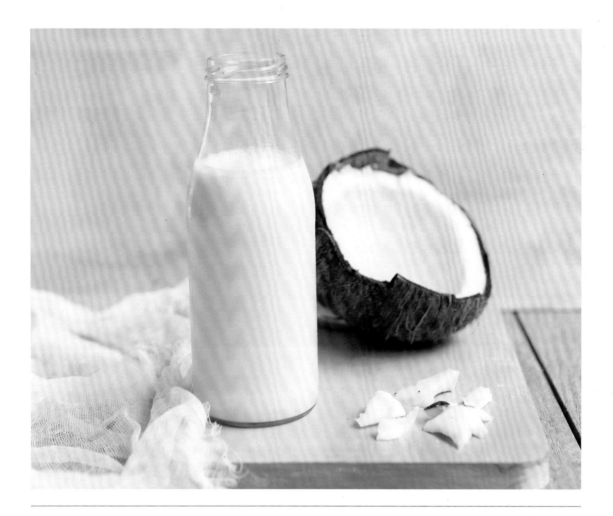

COCONUT MILK

4 cups filtered water
2 cups shredded coconut
   nut milk bag

Heat the water until almost boiling. Place the coconut and heated water into the blender. Blend on high until smooth. Strain the coconut milk through the nut milk bag and then transfer to an airtight container (I suggest mason jars). Refrigerate and use within three days. Shake well before using.

Tip: USE THIS SIMPLE AND EASY HOMEMADE RECIPE INSTEAD OF BUYING THE CANNED OR BOXED COCONUT MILK THAT IS FULL OF UNHEALTHY PRESERVATIVES AND ADDITIVES.

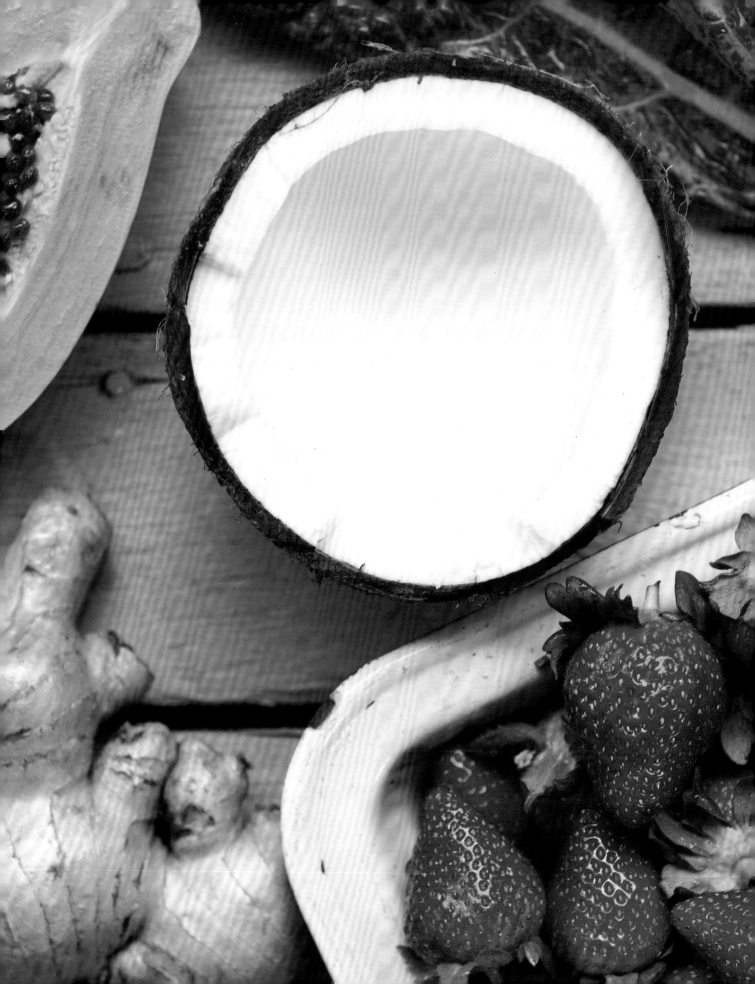

SWEET HAZELNUT MILK

1 cup hazelnut milk
(see 'Nut Milk —
unsweetened' recipe,
page 59)

2 medjool dates

Add the ingredients to a blender.
Blend and enjoy!

ENERGY BOOSTER SMOOTHIE

1 banana, fresh or preferably
frozen

1 cup almond milk (see
'Almond Milk — unsweetened'
recipe, page 58)

1 tablespoon almond butter

1 cup frozen berries
(blackberries, blueberries
and/or raspberries)

1 teaspoon maca powder
(Peruvian ginseng)

1 teaspoon ground chia seeds

1 handful cacao nibs

Peel the banana and cut in half. Add
all the ingredients to the blender.
Blend and enjoy!

Tip: SOME ATHLETES USE
MACA POWDER TO INCREASE
STAMINA. OTHER PEOPLE USE
IT TO BOOST LIBIDO AND
INCREASE FERTILITY!

FULL OF NUTS SMOOTHIE

1 handful cashews

1 banana, fresh or preferably
frozen

¼ pineapple, fresh or preferably
frozen

1 cup almond milk (see
'Almond Milk — unsweetened'
recipe, page 58)

1 medjool date

Soak the cashews in water for 2
hours. Peel the banana and cut in
half. Peel the pineapple and cut into
pieces. Add all the ingredients to the
blender. Blend and enjoy!

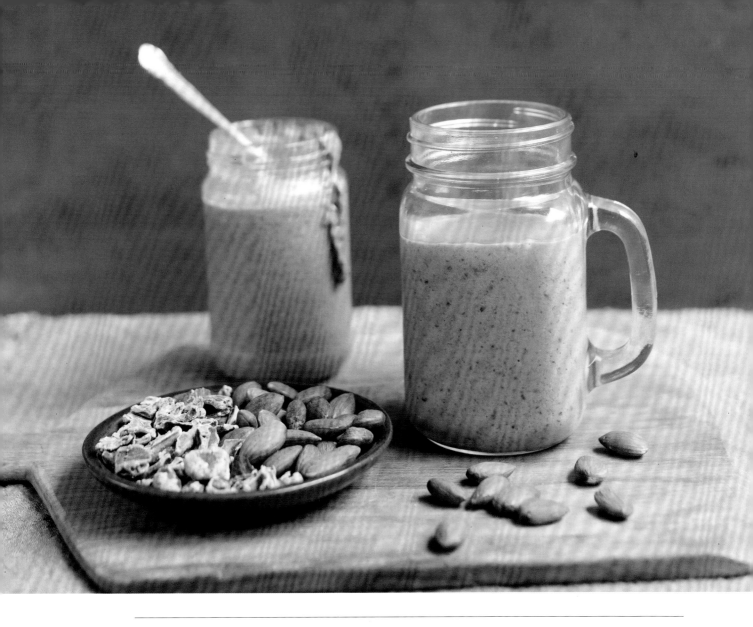

DOUBLE ALMOND SMOOTHIE

1   banana, fresh or preferably
    frozen
1   cup almond milk (see
    'Almond Milk — unsweetened'
    recipe, page 58)
1   tablespoon cacao nibs
1   tablespoon ABC (almond,
    Brazil nut, cashew) butter
1   teaspoon coconut nectar
    pinch of cinnamon

Peel the banana and cut in half. Add
all the ingredients to the blender.
Blend and enjoy!

COCONUT HEMP SMOOTHIE

1 banana, fresh or preferably frozen

1 cup coconut water

1 cup frozen berries (blackberries, blueberries and/or raspberries)

2 tablespoons hemp protein

1 teaspoon coconut oil

Peel the banana and cut in half. Add all the ingredients to the blender. Blend and enjoy!

ALMOND NECTAR PROTEIN SMOOTHIE

1 banana, fresh or preferably frozen

1 cup almond milk (see 'Almond Milk — unsweetened' recipe, page 58)

1 teaspoon ABC (almond, Brazil nut and cashew) butter

1 teaspoon coconut nectar

1 tablespoon protein powder (pea, brown rice)

pinch of cinnamon

Peel the banana and cut in half. Add the banana, almond milk, ABC butter, coconut nectar and protein powder to the blender. Blend. Sprinkle with a dash of cinnamon and enjoy!

REAL COCONUT SMOOTHIE

1 banana, fresh or preferably frozen

½ cup coconut water

½ cup almond or nut milk (see 'Almond Milk — unsweetened' recipe, page 58, or 'Nut Milk — unsweetened' recipe, page 59)

2 medjool dates

1 tablespoon shredded coconut

Peel the banana and cut in half. Add all the ingredients to the blender. Blend and enjoy!

CHOCOLATE CHERRY SMOOTHIE

1 banana, fresh or preferably frozen

1 cup nut milk (see 'Nut Milk — unsweetened' recipe, page 59)

1 teaspoon coconut oil

1 teaspoon almond butter

1 handful cacao chips

1 teaspoon ground chia seeds

1 cup cherries, fresh or preferably frozen

1 cup blackberries, fresh or preferably frozen

Peel the banana and cut in half. Add all the ingredients to the blender. Blend and enjoy!

CACAO SMOOTHIE

1 banana, fresh or preferably frozen

1 cup almond milk (see 'Almond Milk — unsweetened' recipe, page 58)

1 tablespoon cacao powder

1 tablespoon cacao nibs

1 teaspoon almond butter

1 teaspoon coconut oil

1 medjool date

pinch of cinnamon

Peel the banana and cut in half. Add the banana, almond milk, cacao powder, cacao nibs, almond butter, coconut oil and date to the blender. Blend. Sprinkle with a dash of cinnamon and enjoy!

SMOOTH COCONUT SMOOTHIE

1 handful almonds or cashews

1 avocado

1 cup coconut water

1 teaspoon cacao powder

Soak the nuts in water for a minimum of 8 hours. Peel and pit the avocado. Add all the ingredients to the blender. Blend and enjoy!

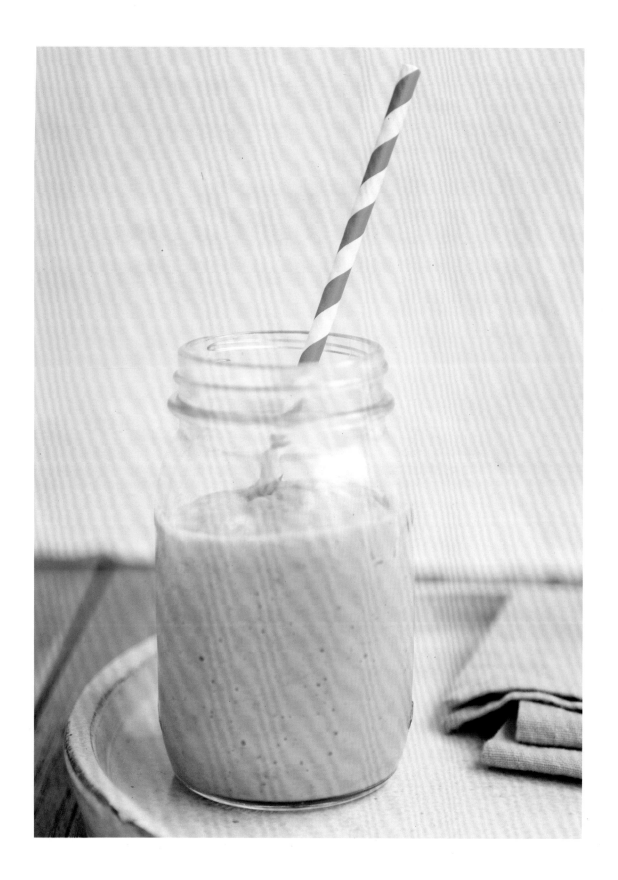

CHLORELLA AND BERRY SMOOTHIE

1   banana, fresh or preferably
     frozen
1   cup filtered water
1   cup frozen berries
     (blackberries, blueberries
     and/or raspberries)
1   tablespoon coconut oil
1   tablespoon (or scoop)
     chlorella powder

Peel the banana and cut in half. Add all the ingredients to the blender. Blend and enjoy!

GREEN PINEAPPLE SMOOTHIE

½   banana, peeled and
     preferably frozen
1   handful cos (romaine) lettuce
½   cucumber
1   stalk silverbeet
¼   avocado
¼   pineapple, fresh or preferably
     frozen
1   cup filtered water

Cut the banana in half. Cut the lettuce, cucumber and silverbeet into pieces. Peel and pit the avocado. Peel the pineapple and cut into pieces. Add all the ingredients to the blender. Blend and enjoy!

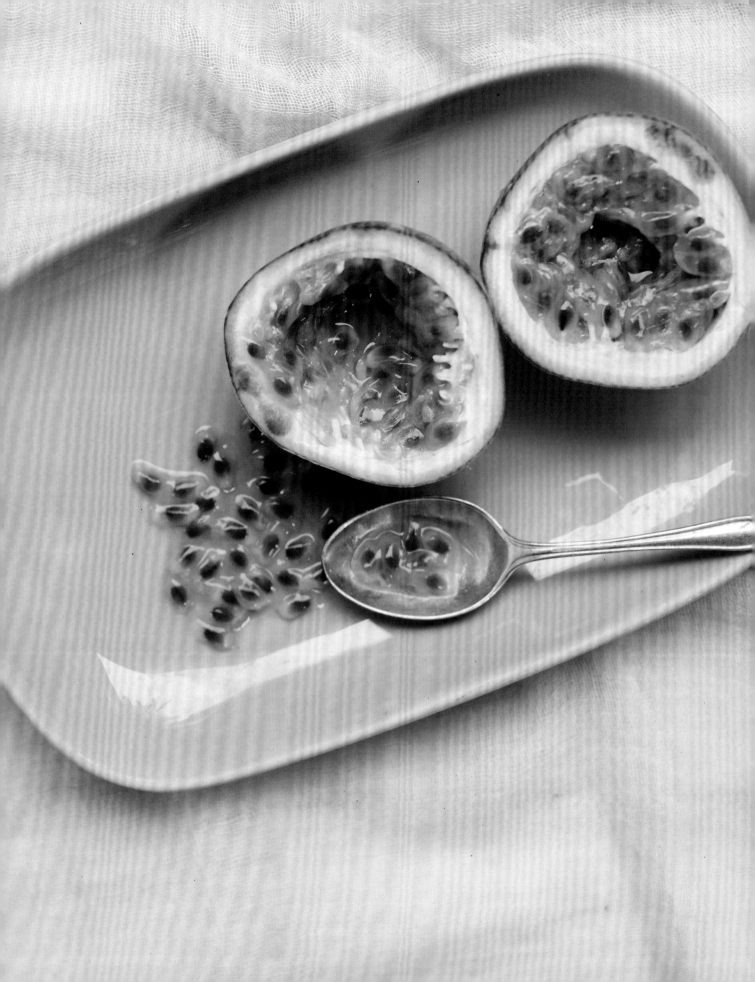

CHAPTER 4

WHOLE FAMILY

Whether you are expecting your first baby or have a small tribe to look after, it's easy to get your whole family on board with juicing. Start gently: try juicing with a few (two or three) fruits and one vegetable to start, and if you have kids try some of the child-friendly recipes because they are an easy way to acclimatize everyone. Use this book to increase vitamin intake all-round, and involve everyone in recipe-tasting. Most of all, enjoy it!

CHILDREN AND JUICING

Juice is for everyone. Yes, that includes kids! My nine-year-old full-of-energy, full-of-love stepson Max loves juices *and* smoothies. In fact, he asks for them every day. Our morning is filled with excited conversation around what I am going to juice for him, what fruit and vegetables he will take to school and what smoothie he will get that afternoon. It brings me so much happiness; in fact, I bought him an apron and he now works alongside me in the kitchen. Yes, that's right: my nine-year-old stepson is a juice lover, recipe taste-tester and all-round healthy boy. In this chapter I have included his favourite recipes, including some we have created together.

When getting started I suggest using two different fruits and one vegetable in juices or smoothies to familiarize your children with the taste. Once they become familiar with vegetables in their juices and smoothies, you can add more. I also suggest using a brightly coloured BPA-free cup (possibly with its own straw, so if or when you do start adding greens, the kids won't be turned off by the colour.

As a rule, try not to use too much fruit in your juices, because the fruit can turn to fructose, leaving your children with a sugar high. If you want to add fruit, the best thing to do is start them off with smoothies, because there is a slow absorption of fruit when the fibre is left in. If you do want to give your children juice, however, I start simply with one of these ingredients: carrots, apples, pears, watermelon or beets. The sweet taste will bring them back for more. Eventually you can add greens, little by little.

Win your kids over by starting them off with smoothies first.

JUICING AND SMOOTHIES WHILE EXPECTING

Speaking of the whole family, while writing *Juice It, Blend It!* I became pregnant with my gorgeous little girl. Actually, on the day I found out I would be writing *Juice It, Blend It!* she was conceived. And, not long after I finished writing this book she arrived. So, she too was a taste-tester, and judging by her daily movements she loved juicing!

During my pregnancy I focused on diet and healthy eating more so than ever. I became obsessed with reducing sugars and learned a lot about everything I was putting into my body. I tested loads of new smoothie options that were healthy and filled with superfoods. I became a research queen on all things plant-based and wanted to incorporate all of this love into her life while she was in the womb. I started adding nectarines to all of my smoothies, and I craved carob nibs, almond butter, nut milks and bananas. And yes, these are healthy additives.

So, if you are looking to fall pregnant, are currently pregnant or breastfeeding, I have some recommendations on yummy smoothies to keep you healthy. In addition, I have shared some vitamins you will need to keep you and your baby healthy.

VITAMINS AND MINERALS NEEDED WHEN YOU ARE EXPECTING AND/OR BREASTFEEDING

Let's start with the vitamins you need and foods to incorporate to get them:

» **Folate (also known as folic acid). Part of the vitamin B family, folate helps protect your baby against birth defects. Add broccoli and spinach to your juices and smoothies for an extra dose.**

» **Iron. Low levels of iron are linked to premature and low-birth-weight babies. However, iron in the plant form requires vitamin C for the best iron absorption, so pair spinach with oranges or tomatoes (or see vitamin C suggestions below).**

» **Vitamin B. Vitamin B is important for your baby's brain and development. Incorporate lots of fruit and vegetables that are high in vitamin B into your diet to ensure you are keeping your baby healthy in the womb: avocado, spinach, bananas, berries, pineapple or passionfruit. Also, dates and hazelnuts are known to be high in vitamin B.**

» **Vitamin C. To supplement vitamin C in your pre-natal diet, add a juice or smoothie with any of the fruit and vegetables that are high in vitamin C, such as: dark leafy greens, strawberries, kiwi, citrus and tomatoes.**

During pregnancy women need a balanced diet, but without added sugars or anything raw or unpasteurized. To best achieve this, know the source. No store-bought sugar- and preservative-filled juices and no raw, unpasteurized juice you get from a healthy juice bar. Basically, make your own juice and make it healthy, ensuring you are getting the right vitamins and minerals.

PASTEURIZED VERSUS UNPASTEURIZED

Pasteurization is the process used to heat and kill bacteria, which also kills the nutrients and enzymes you are looking to get from vegetables. When a food is unpasteurized, it is left untreated and therefore can harbour bacteria that can be dangerous during pregnancy. When making your juice at home, clean your fruit and vegetables well (see my tips on page 20); you can even do a home flash-pasteurization by boiling water and pouring it over your fruit and vegetables. Additionally, drink the juice within three to four minutes after making it.

Tip: IT IS UNSAFE TO DEEP CLEANSE OR DETOX IN PREGNANCY OR WHILE BREASTFEEDING.

Some things to think about adding to your juices and/or smoothies while you are pregnant:

First trimester, when you will possibly battle nausea and fatigue: ginger, orange, apple, dark leafy greens.

Second and third trimesters, when you will possibly battle heartburn (also known as acid reflux), constipation, foot and leg cramps, sinus congestion, back pain and fatigue, and might be diagnosed with gestational diabetes and/or iron deficiency: mint, leafy greens, spinach, broccoli, bananas, coconut water, nuts, nut milks and vitamin C powerhouse superfoods.

Tip: AN APPLE A DAY IS SAID TO KEEP ASTHMA AWAY FROM UNBORN BABIES.

JUICY RECIPES

GOOD MORNING SUNSHINE FOR THE WHOLE GANG

3 carrots
1 apple (gala or green)

Cut the tips off the carrots. Cut the apple to fit into the juicer. Feed the ingredients through the juicer. Pour into a glass and serve immediately. Enjoy!

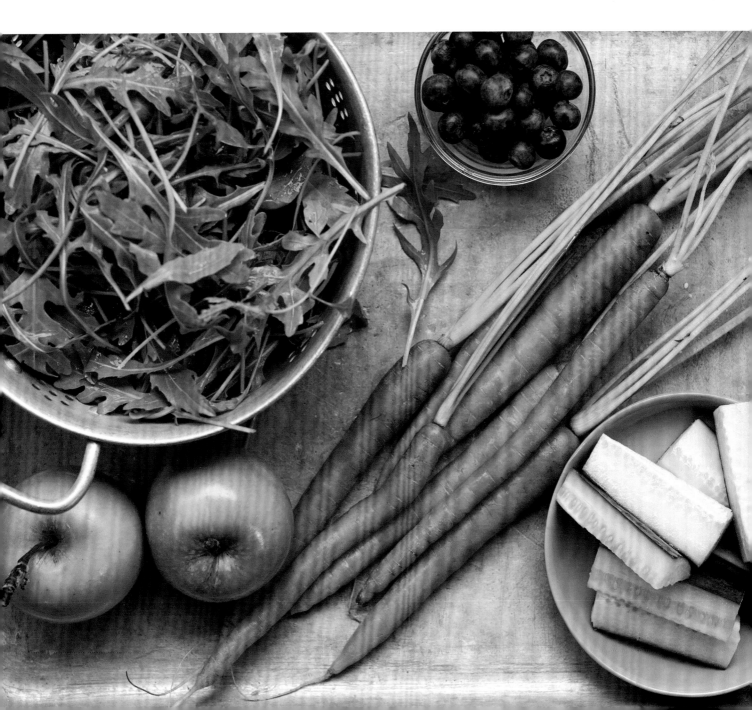

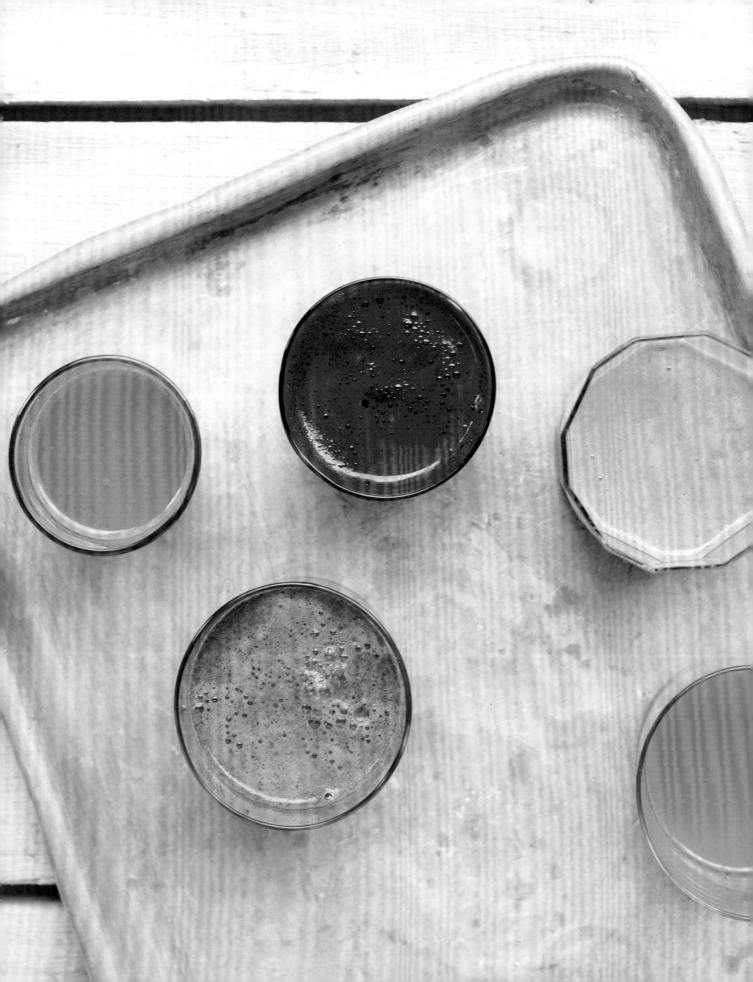

VITAMIN C AND LEAFY GREENS JUICE

2 carrots
1 apple
1 handful spinach
1 tomato

Cut the tips off the carrots. Cut the apple to fit into the juicer. Feed the ingredients through the juicer. Pour into a glass and serve immediately. Enjoy!

IRON-RICH JUICE FOR MOTHERS AND KIDS

1 large orange
2 handfuls spinach

Peel and remove the pith from the orange and then cut in half. Feed the ingredients through the juicer. Pour into a glass and serve immediately. Enjoy!

APPLE AND ORANGE JUICE

2 oranges
2 apples

Peel and remove the pith from the oranges and then cut them in half. Cut the apples to fit into the juicer. Feed the ingredients through the juicer. Pour into a glass and serve immediately. Enjoy!

FRUIT FANTASTIC FOR BEGINNER JUICERS

2 carrots
1 orange
1 pear

Cut the tips off the carrots. Peel and remove the pith from the orange and then cut in half. Cut the pear to fit into the juicer. Feed the ingredients through the juicer. Pour into a glass and serve immediately. Enjoy!

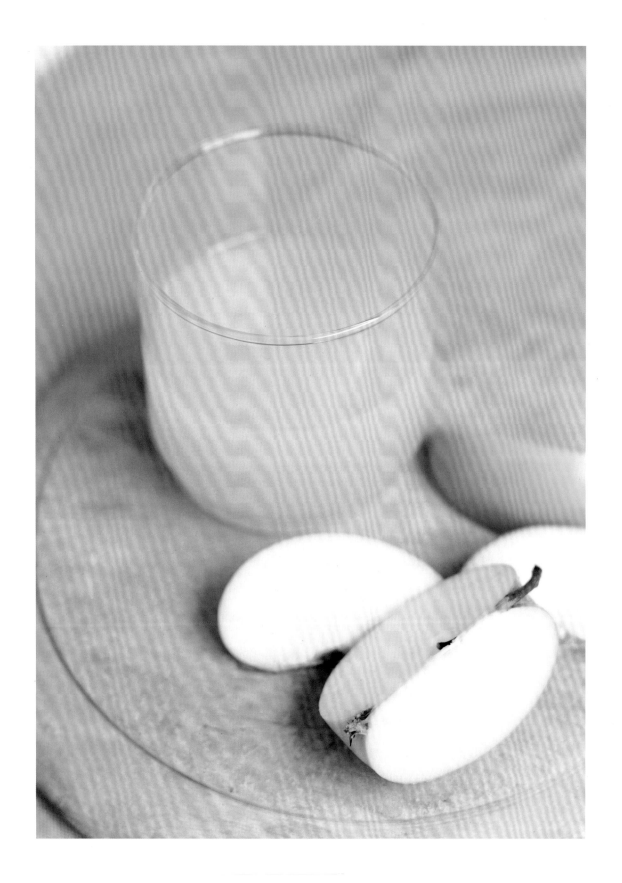

KIDS-LOVE-VEGETABLES JUICE

2 carrots
1 handful spinach
1 tomato
1 cucumber
½ lemon

Cut the tips off the carrots. Feed the carrots, spinach, tomato and cucumber through the juicer. Pour into a glass. Using your citrus reamer, squeeze the lemon directly into your juice. Serve immediately. Enjoy!

MAMA JUICE

2 apples
1 knob ginger
1 lemon
1 sprig thyme

Cut the apples to fit into the juicer. Feed the apples and ginger through the juicer. Pour into a glass. Using your citrus reamer, squeeze the lemon directly into your juice. Add the thyme as a topping. Serve immediately. Enjoy!

GINGER NAUSEA AIDE

2 apples
3 stalks celery
1 knob ginger

Cut the apples to fit into the juicer. Feed the ingredients through the juicer. Pour into a glass and serve immediately. Enjoy!

ANTENATAL PUNCH JUICE

1 beet
1 handful kale
1 handful spinach

Cut the beet to fit into the juicer. Feed all the ingredients through the juicer. Pour into a glass and serve immediately. Enjoy!

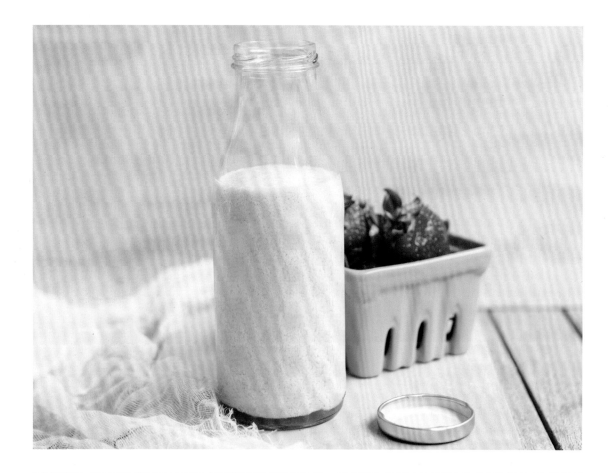

STRAWBERRY ALMOND MILK

½ banana, fresh or preferably
frozen

1 cup almond milk (see
'Almond Milk — unsweetened'
recipe, page 58)

½ cup strawberries, hulled and
fresh or frozen

Peel the banana and cut in half. Add
all the ingredients to the blender.
Blend and enjoy!

CACAO ALMOND MILK

1 cup almond milk (see
'Almond Milk — unsweetened'
recipe, page 58)

1 tablespoon cacao powder

Add all the ingredients to a blender.
Blend and enjoy!

KALE AND PINEAPPLE SMOOTHIE

1   carrot
½   cucumber
½   apple
¼   pineapple
1   banana, fresh or preferably frozen
1   cup filtered water
1   handful kale
½   lemon
1   handful blackberries, fresh or frozen

Cut the tip off the carrot. Cut the carrot, cucumber and apple into small pieces. Peel the pineapple and cut into pieces. Peel the banana and cut in half. Add all the ingredients to the blender. Blend and enjoy!

STRAWBERRY MANGO BANANA SMOOTHIE

1   banana, fresh or preferably frozen
1   mango, fresh or frozen
1   cup coconut water
1   cup strawberries, hulled and fresh or frozen

Peel the banana and cut in half. Remove the pit from the mango and then cut the flesh into pieces. Add all the ingredients to the blender. Blend and enjoy!

CLEAN GREEN SMOOTHIE

1   banana, fresh or preferably frozen
1   handful spinach
1   cup almond milk (see 'Almond Milk – unsweetened' recipe, page 58)
1   tablespoon spirulina powder
½   lime

Peel the banana and cut in half. Cut the spinach into pieces. Add the banana, spinach, almond milk and spirulina to the blender. Blend. Using a citrus reamer, squeeze the lime directly into the smoothie. Enjoy!

NECTARINE SMOOTHIE

1   nectarine, fresh or
    frozen
1   banana, fresh or preferably
    frozen
1   cup almond milk (see
    'Almond Milk — unsweetened'
    recipe, page 58)
1   handful fresh mint
1   tablespoon ABC (almond,
    Brazil nut, cashew) butter

Remove the pit from the nectarine
and then cut the flesh into pieces.
Peel the banana and cut in half. Add
all the ingredients to the blender.
Blend and enjoy!

KIDS LOVE JUICE AND SMOOTHIE MIX

1   cup orange juice (using
    freshly juiced oranges)
1   banana, fresh or preferably
    frozen
1   cup strawberries, hulled

Peel the oranges and remove the
pith, then cut in half and juice in
a juicer. Add the orange juice to
the blender. Peel the banana and
cut in half. Add the banana and
strawberries to the blender. Blend and
enjoy!

RASPBERRY CACAO SMOOTHIE

1   cup almond milk (see
    'Almond Milk — unsweetened'
    recipe, page 58)
2   cups raspberries, frozen
1   teaspoon almond butter
1   teaspoon cacao powder
1   teaspoon cacao nibs
    (to add as topping)

Add the almond milk, raspberries,
almond butter and cacao powder
to the blender. Blend. Top with the
cacao nibs and enjoy!

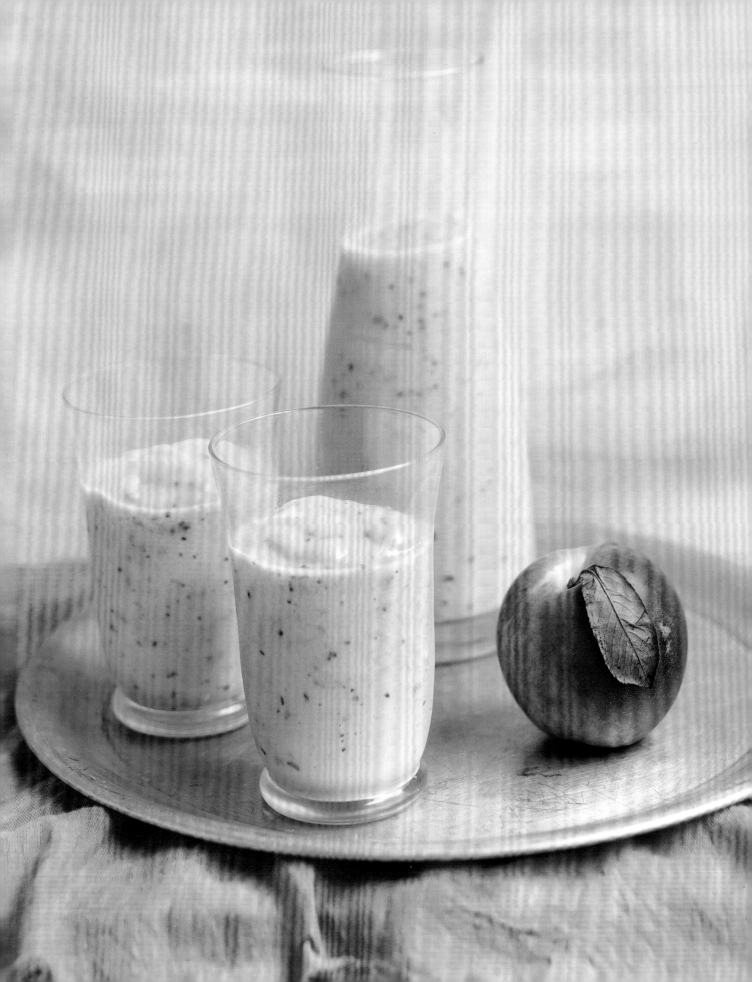

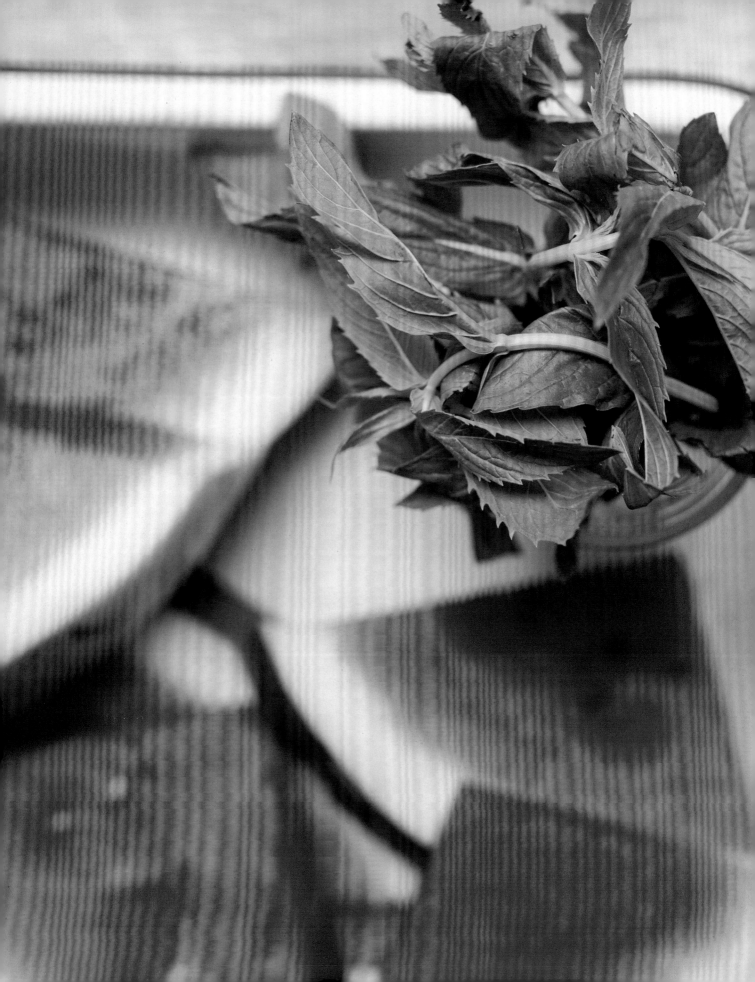

CHAPTER 5

RELAX

Do you ever feel overwhelmed? Overworked? Anxious? Stressed? These days everyone seems to be overwhelmed, overworked, anxious and stressed. We are always in a rush, always working to a deadline and moving on to the next thing. It seems natural to have a busy schedule with little down time, and even when we do take some time out we fill it with television or external habits that don't support our overall wellbeing. I sometimes find myself not living in the moment; I think about what happened yesterday or what is on my to-do list for tomorrow. I share overwhelming lists with my husband, who laughs and tells me to just take time out and breathe.

Stress has a negative effect on our emotional wellbeing and physical body. Stress overworks the adrenal glands and produces two hormones called cortisol and DHEA, which are the root cause of the extra weight around the waistline. Many people tell me they are doing everything they can to keep fit but just can't get rid of the weight. When I learn about their stressful lifestyle or work habits it is very clear where the weight is coming from: stress.

So, how do you combat stress? First, start your morning off right. Then, have an afternoon routine that keeps you healthy. Look after yourself and don't burn the candle at both ends. Oh, and of course JUICE!

Juices and smoothies can help you to fight stress.

TIPS TO REDUCE STRESS

Start with some of my tips and end with a healthy juice or smoothie to wind down:

- » **Burn candles.**

- » **Listen to calming music.**

- » **Discover cupping and acupuncture. Together they are mind-blowing. I always feel extremely relaxed, calm and balanced after a session. Cupping pulls the toxins and bad energy from your body through suction created on the skin, using glass and fire (although there are other methods and techniques, this is my personal favourite). I suggest doing your research to find someone that specializes in traditional Chinese medicine, and have acupuncture and cupping done together, by a licensed professional.**

- » **Use essential oils. Burn beautiful scented oils in your home: my favourites are lavender, rose and jasmine.**

- » **Go for a massage. I suggest a massage at least once a month. I love a 60-minute aromatherapy massage with oils to bring you to deep relaxation.**

- » **Meditate. Let stillness become who you are. Create stories in your mind and build upon them; your stories become your reality. In order to be in the moment and not become the stories you create in your mind look at nature and be in the moment. Find the method of meditation that's right for you.**

- » **Breathe. Try different breathing techniques to calm your mind and body. I suggest breathing in through your nose and then out from your tummy (in an outward motion).**

- » **Move! Try walking, or simply getting up and moving around. Moving is your friend. Boost your circulation and release endorphins!**

- » **Scrub. This is my secret weapon. Whenever I feel anxious I jump in the shower and scrub the thoughts and dead skin** away. It is super easy to make your own scrub; one of my favourites is a mix of ¼ cup coconut or olive oil, ½ cup brown sugar and a dash of essential oil (lemon, rose or your favourite scent) stored in a mason jar.

» Step out in the sunlight. Just twenty minutes in the morning or afternoon for a dose of vitamin D.

» Yoga. To me, yoga is a state of mind. To some, yoga is a physical form. I believe that once you find balance you will learn how to calm your system, and yoga is a way to help you achieve this. Using the body to calm the mind is a beautiful thing.

» Take a warm bath. Try adding Epsom salts and rose petals to a warm running bath. Grab your favourite book, dim the lights and indulge.

» Make a smoothie relaxer. Anything we put into our body can affect the way we handle anxiety and stress. When you choose sugary foods and drinks over healthy plant food your body knows the difference. Instead of feeding your body harmful ingredients, why not load up on stuff that makes your body and mind feel good?

HEALING SMOOTHIE ADDITIVES

Let's dive into some amazing healing foods that can help you remain calm, balanced and centred.

» Blackberries are a great dose of fibre and folate, and they are also known to help reduce the effects of mood disorders. All berries are full of antioxidants, but blackberries take the cake, so adding them to your smoothies is a no-brainer.

» Bananas help lift your mood and shake the blues. This is because bananas are filled with vitamins A, B6 and C as well as fibre, potassium and healthy carbohydrates. A mood-lifting powerhouse!

» Cacao is the ideal, delicious alternative when you crave a sweet treat to boost your mood.

» Celery can help lower stress hormones in the blood, helping your body to stress less!

» Leafy greens such as kale and spinach are rich in vitamin B and a great mood enhancer.

JUICY RECIPES

CELERY CALMER

1 small tomato
4 stalks celery
½ cucumber
1 handful coriander (cilantro)

Cut the tomato to fit into the juicer. Feed the ingredients through the juicer. Pour into a glass and serve immediately. Enjoy!

BROCCOLI KALE PARSLEY JUICE

1 apple
2 broccoli florets
1 handful kale
2 stalks celery
1 handful parsley

Cut the apple to fit into the juicer. Feed the ingredients through the juicer. Pour into a glass and serve immediately. Enjoy!

GRAPEFRUIT KALE JUICE

1 grapefruit
1 handful kale
1 cucumber

Cut the grapefruit in half, then peel and remove the pith, and cut the grapefruit to fit into the juicer. Feed the ingredients through the juicer. Pour into a glass and serve immediately. Enjoy!

PURPLE KALE SMOOTHIE

½ cucumber
1 handful kale
1 cup coconut water
1 cup blackberries, fresh or preferably frozen

Cut the cucumber and kale into small pieces. Add all the ingredients to a blender. Blend and enjoy!

BEATING THE BLUES SMOOTHIE

1 banana, fresh or preferably frozen
1 teaspoon ground chia seeds
1 cup almond milk (see 'Almond Milk — unsweetened' recipe, page 58)
1 cup blackberries, fresh or preferably frozen
1 small handful cacao nibs
1 teaspoon spirulina powder

Peel the banana and cut in half. Use a food processor to ground the chia seeds (or leave them whole). Add all the ingredients to a blender. Blend and enjoy!

GOING NUTS FOR GREENS SMOOTHIE

1 handful spinach
1 banana, fresh or preferably frozen
1 cup hazelnut milk (see 'Nut Milk — unsweetened' recipe, page 59)
1 handful cacao nibs
2 medjool dates
  pinch of cinnamon

Cut the spinach into small pieces. Peel the banana and cut in half. Add the spinach, banana, hazelnut milk, cacao nibs and dates to the blender. Blend. Pour into a glass and add a pinch of cinnamon. Enjoy!

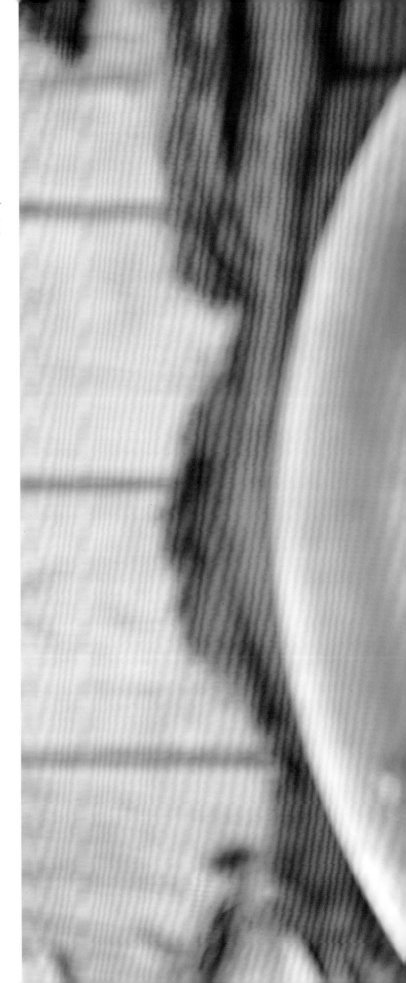

CALMING ROSE SMOOTHIE

1   banana, fresh or preferably
    frozen
½   cup strawberries, fresh or
    preferably frozen
½   cup coconut milk
    (see 'Coconut Milk' recipe,
    page 60)
½   cup coconut or filtered water
¼   teaspoon rose water
    edible flowers for topping

Peel the banana and cut in half. Hull
the strawberries. Add the banana,
strawberries, coconut milk, coconut
or filtered water and rose water to a
blender. Blend. Pour into a glass and
top with the gorgeous edible flowers.
Enjoy!

Tip: HAVE THIS
CALMING ROSE SMOOTHIE
WITH YOUR FAVOURITE BOOK
AND PUT YOUR FEET UP. YOU
DESERVE IT!

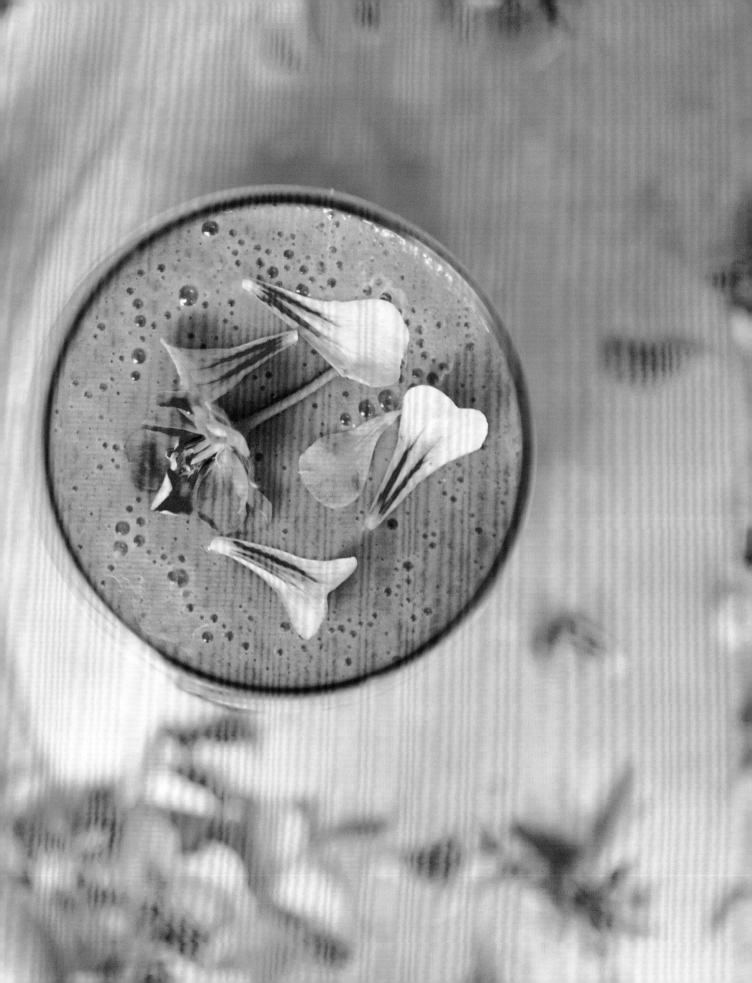

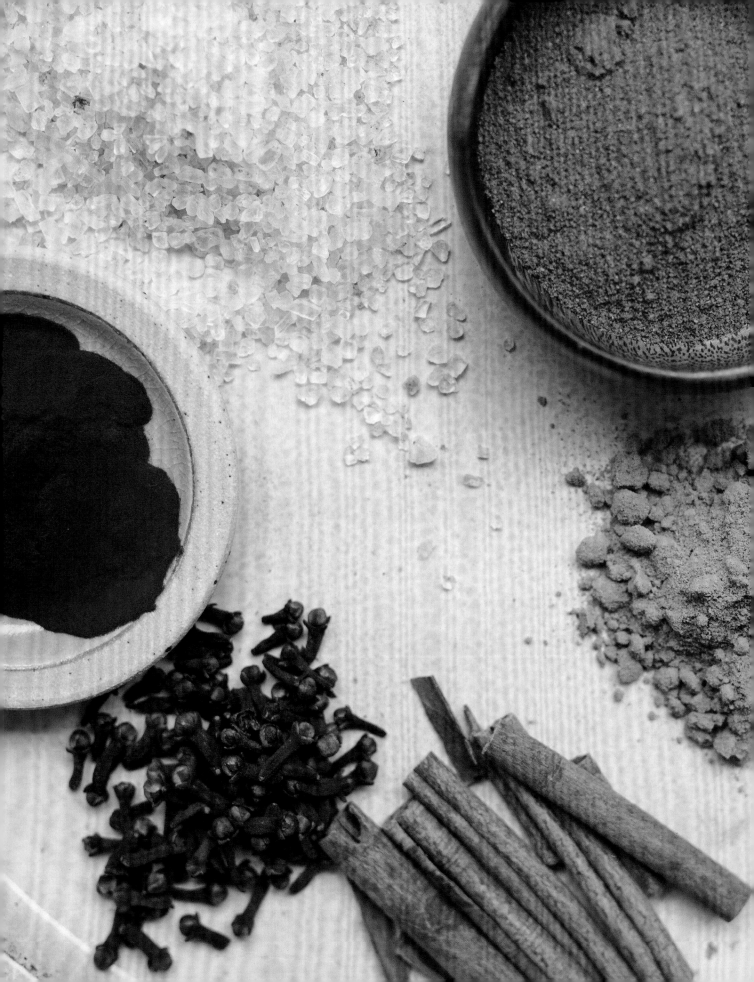

CHAPTER 6

IMMUNITY

When we lack nutrients we gain weight and get sick and tired. That is because our body needs chlorophyll, vitamins and minerals to keep healthy. According to Harvard University's School of Public Health, a diet that is high in fruit and vegetables can lower blood pressure, reduce heart disease and stroke, and could prevent cancer. Choosing fruit and vegetables over processed food could also have a positive effect on our blood sugar levels that in turn keep weight in check.

Including an abundance of plant food in our diet is one of the keys to health.

Choosing plant food means saying goodbye to toxins, stubborn weight gain and sugar addictions, and hello to good energy, feeling healthy, great skin and hello to a happy digestion, all while helping to prevent disease.

Juicing has become popular as a way to heal. For those with severe illnesses who need to absorb the vitamins and nutrients of plant food but can't eat all the required vegetables, juicing can be the answer. This way the body doesn't have to digest as much, but still gets all the benefits of the vitamins and minerals.

BENEFITS OF PLANT FOODS

Let's explore vitamins and minerals and some of the beautiful plant food that is easily accessible and delicious, and also the wonderful array of fruit, vegetables and supplements that will help maintain a healthy immune system.

VITAMINS AND MINERALS

» Calcium is needed for strong bones and healthy function of the heart and muscles. The body doesn't produce calcium on its own, so we need to eat the right foods to ensure we have enough. Some sources include dark leafy greens, broccoli, nuts and silica powder.

» Chromium helps our body metabolize carbohydrates, protein and fat. This mineral can be found in broccoli, apples, oranges, basil and bananas.

» Folate, together with vitamin B12, helps us produce red blood cells. Folate, also known as folic acid, can be found in dark leafy green vegetables, fruit and nuts.

» Iron helps to carry oxygen from our lungs to the rest of our body. Without iron we could be anemic and suffer fatigue and exhaustion. Sources include spinach and nuts.

» Magnesium is a mineral with many benefits. Our body needs magnesium for the proper function of the kidneys, muscles, healthy digestive track and cardiovascular system and brain. It has been said that magnesium supports many health conditions such as constipation, asthma, heart disease as well as some auto-immune disorders such as multiple sclerosis and lupus. Some sources include almonds, avocado, cashews, spinach, carrots and apples.

» Selenium supports our metabolism. A major source is Brazil nuts.

» Vitamin A is essential, but too much vitamin A can be dangerous. The best way to take vitamin A is through food. It is amazing for our immune system and our vision. Some sources include sweet potatoes, spinach, carrots, mango and capsicum (pepper).

» Vitamin B6 is very important, and helps break down protein in our body. Sources include banana, nuts, spinach, watermelon and other fruit (other then citrus).

» Vitamin B12 is hard to get through the absorption of food, so supplements are needed. This powerful nutrient keeps our cells healthy. A supplement source is spirulina in its powder form, although mixed controversial information exists.

» Vitamin D is necessary for our body to absorb calcium. So, get out and soak up the sun for twenty minutes every day. Plant food sources are limited, but you can get what you need soaking up some rays.

» Vitamin E is important for our skin, eyes and overall healthy immune system. Some sources include nuts, oils and nut butters.

» Vitamin K supports strong bones and a healthy heart while helping our blood to clot. A vital source includes spinach, although it could be dangerous if taken with certain medications. Check with your doctor if you are taking blood thinner medications.

» Vitamin C supports the immune system. Some studies have found that vitamin C is effective in killing cancer cells. It has also been said that patients undergoing chemotherapy could see fewer side effects when incorporating high volumes of vitamin C into their system. Some sources of vitamin C include spinach and citrus fruits.

FRUITS, VEGETABLES AND SUPPLEMENTS

» Beets are a powerhouse cleansing, blood-boosting vegetable. They have traces of vitamins and minerals that provide iron, folate, potassium, magnesium and vitamin C to our immune system. Beets are also known for their anti-inflammatory properties.

» Carrots are full of B vitamins, vitamin C and K. They also have a high concentration of vitamin A. These vegetables are a true powerhouse helping our vision and overall immunity!

» Cayenne pepper gives us vitamin A. Add this as a pinch to a citrus juice and you will feel the heat!

» Celery is high in folate and can also provide calcium and magnesium. Try celery in a juice while scooping in spirulina powder. Yum and so healthy!

» Citrus fruits are full of vitamin C, which fully supports our immune system and helps us fight off colds, flu and disease. Nature works in wonderful ways: just when flu season comes on, citrus fruits come in season. Try orange, grapefruit, lemon and lime.

» Coconut water is filled with potassium and magnesium. It is great for hydration and staying healthy.

» Coriander (cilantro) is filled with vitamins. If you like the taste, add it to any juice. I love adding this herb to green juices, especially anything with leafy greens. Coriander is also known to combat mercury in the body and remove toxins. Another reason to love this herb!

» Ginger is an anti-inflammatory and amazing to battle nausea. It's filled with potassium too, so add this to your juices. It is especially yummy in green juices and gives a beautiful kick.

Fruit and vegetables are our natural medicine chest, bursting with vitamins and minerals!

» Kale was once a staple for sheep, but is now seen as a must for all of us. It's a powerhouse vegetable filled with vitamins A, C and K, calcium and folate. I suggest juicing kale a few times a week. I love switching up kale and spinach.

» Parsley cleanses our blood and is filled with vitamin K, among other vitamins and minerals such as folate.

» Spinach has a long list of health benefits. It is filled with vitamins A, B, C, E and K, iron and much more.

» Spirulina is a superfood filled with chlorophyll, iron and vitamin B12, and is a must juice or smoothie additive. Give this a try and feel the juicy effects.

» Wheatgrass is known to combat disease, fatigue and gray hair! It is full of iron, calcium, magnesium and chlorophyll.

Your digestive system is working hard ... so, remember to always juice at least two or three hours after eating to allow the vitamins and minerals to go straight to your bloodstream. Juice gets into your blood system within twenty minutes. Wait 30 minutes before eating after a juice. Digestion is key and knowing when to juice and eat right will make a difference.

SOME OTHER TIPS TO SAVE YOUR IMMUNE SYSTEM

» Juice and blend with the seasons, and always choose local produce. If you decide to freeze fruit, buy in season, make sure it's ripe, and store in your freezer.

» Do you have a nut allergy? Choose coconut milk. Don't want to choose an alternative milk-based product? Choose coconut water or filtered water!

» Buy a filter to keep filtered water accessible in your home. I recommend an alkaline water filter. Do your research, but note that the better the water tastes, the better the benefits and the more you will drink!

» Buy a glass jar and take your alkaline filtered water on the go!

» There are health risks associated with artificial sweeteners; these chemicals should be avoided and never added to your juices or smoothies.

»   I never use store-bought fruit juice in my smoothies. And, I never add sugar (see options for natural sweeteners on page 54). Instead of store-bought fruit juice, make it yourself and then add it to your smoothie so you know the sugar content.

»   If you are young, elderly or ill, you should choose organic fruit and vegetables. Always.

»   If you are taking medication, always consult with your doctor in case you need to restrict your ingredients.

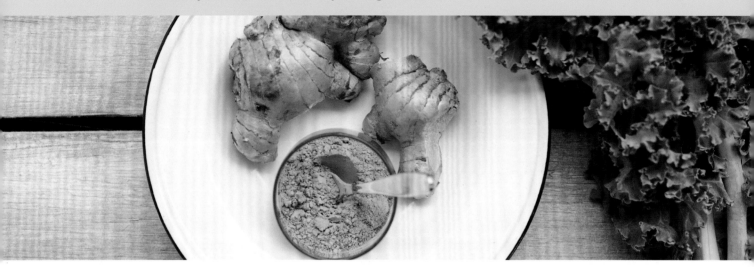

JUICY ADDITIVES

There are some amazing superfoods you can add to your already healthy juices. Here are some of my favourites!

CHLORELLA POWDER

Juice and smoothie addition
One of the most widely researched foods, chlorella (or chlorophyll) is a green superfood that supports our immune system and contains loads of vitamins and minerals.

Juice additive: Once you have juiced your ingredients, stir in your powder and drink up.

Smoothie additive: Add 1 teaspoon to your daily smoothie with all the ingredients and blend.

MACA POWDER

Smoothie addition

Maca is a superfood that some think is a miracle worker. Also known as Peruvian ginseng, it's full of vitamins like B, C and E. It's also full of minerals like calcium, iron, magnesium and zinc. It has been said to improve sexual function and women's moods and energy. I've seen maca sold in pill form, but I love it as part of my smoothie. It's tasteless, but I know it's supporting me.

Smoothie additive: Add 1 teaspoon to your daily smoothie with all the ingredients and blend.

SPIRULINA

Juice and smoothie addition

This superfood is filled with loads of necessary vitamins and minerals. Spirulina is a green powder super high in chlorophyll.

Juice additive: Once you have juiced your ingredients, stir in your powder and drink up.

Smoothie additive: Add 1 teaspoon to your daily smoothie with all the ingredients and blend.

WHEATGRASS POWDER

Juice and smoothie addition

Wheatgrass, similar to chlorophyll, is full of vitamins and minerals. It is a fabulous way to add all of your daily green vegetables to your diet. Add 1 teaspoon (to start, but once you are comfortable and feel that you can handle more try up to 1 tablespoon) to any of your juices or smoothies.

Juice additive: Once you have juiced your ingredients, stir in your powder and drink up.

Smoothie additive: Add 1 teaspoon to your daily smoothie with all the ingredients and blend.

JUICY RECIPES

POMEGRANATE POWER JUICE

1 pomegranate
1½ apples

Cut the pomegranate in half and remove the arils (seeds). Cut the apples to fit into the juicer. Feed the ingredients through the juicer. Pour into a glass and serve immediately. Enjoy!

VITAMIN C HEALER

2 carrots
1 handful kale
¼ green capsicum (pepper)
1 handful parsley
1 knob ginger

Cut the tips off the carrots. Feed the ingredients through the juicer. Pour into a glass and serve immediately. Enjoy!

ALL GREENS HEALER JUICE

1 green apple
2 kale leaves
½ cucumber
1 handful spinach
1 sprig parsley
½ lime

Cut the apple to fit into the juicer. Feed the apple, kale, cucumber, spinach and parsley through the juicer. Pour into a glass. Using your citrus reamer, squeeze the lime directly into your juice. Serve immediately. Try stirring in 1 teaspoon of spirulina powder, chlorella or wheatgrass to add some vitamins and minerals. Enjoy!

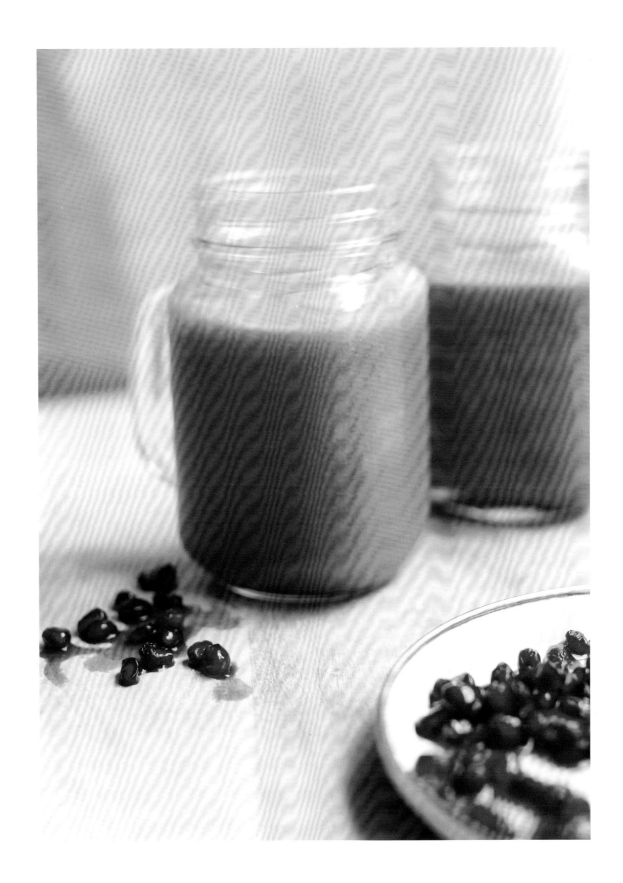

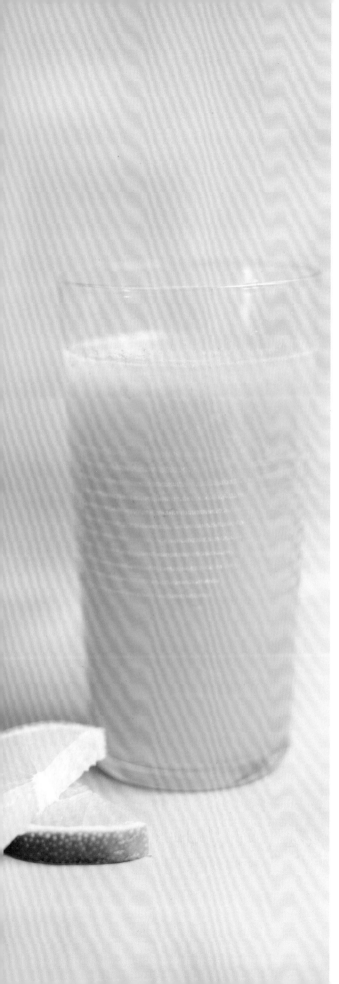

BITTER CELERY JUICE

1 green apple
2 stalks celery
1 handful rocket (arugula)
1 green apple
1 knob ginger
½ lime, peel on

Cut the apple to fit into the juicer.
Feed all the ingredients through the
juicer. Pour into a glass and serve
immediately. Try stirring in 1 teaspoon
of spirulina powder, chlorella or
wheatgrass to add some vitamins and
minerals. Enjoy!

Tip: THE PEEL OF LEMONS
AND LIMES IS FILLED WITH
ANTI-OXIDANTS AND CAN
REDUCE CHOLESTEROL.
HOWEVER, IT ISN'T EASY ON
THE STOMACH. YOU CAN
DIGEST AS MUCH AS HALF A
PEEL A DAY BEFORE GETTING A
TUMMY ACHE. GO FOR IT!

ORANGE JUICE

3 oranges

Remove the peel and pith from the oranges and cut in half. Feed the oranges through the juicer. Pour into a glass and serve immediately. Enjoy!

Tip: REMOVE THE PEEL AND PITH OF AN ORANGE BECAUSE THE PEEL HAS OIL THAT CAN CAUSE INDIGESTION. AS WE ARE TALKING ABOUT IMMUNITY I THINK IT IS IMPORTANT TO LOOK AFTER YOUR HEALTH! I HAVE TRIED JUICING WITH THE PEEL ON, BUT I DO NOT RECOMMEND IT!

MINTY LOVE JUICE

1 handful kale
2 stalks celery
1 small bunch mint
1 sprig parsley
½ cucumber
½ lemon

Feed all the ingredients through the juicer. Pour into a glass and serve immediately. Try stirring in 1 teaspoon of spirulina powder, chlorella or wheatgrass to add some vitamins and minerals. Enjoy!

FENNEL AND KALE JUICE

1 bulb fennel
1 apple
1 handful kale
1 cucumber
1 handful mint
½ lemon

Cut the fennel and apple to fit into the juicer. Feed all the ingredients through the juicer. Pour into a glass and serve immediately. Try stirring in 1 teaspoon of spirulina powder, chlorella or wheatgrass to add some vitamins and minerals. Enjoy!

SWEET DANDELION JUICE

1 pear
1 handful kale
½ cucumber
1 handful dandelion
1 lime

Cut the pear to fit into the juicer. Feed the pear, kale, cucumber and dandelion through the juicer. Pour into a glass. Using your citrus reamer, squeeze the lime directly into your juice. Serve immediately. Try stirring in 1 teaspoon of spirulina powder, chlorella or wheatgrass to add some vitamins and minerals. Enjoy!

CARROT JUICE

6 carrots

Cut the tips off the carrots. Feed the carrots through the juicer. Pour into a glass and serve immediately. Enjoy!

PEAR GINGER JUICE

2 pears
1 knob ginger

Cut the pears to fit into the juicer. Feed the pears and ginger through the juicer. Pour into a glass and serve immediately. Enjoy!

ORANGE CORIANDER JUICE

2 oranges
1 handful coriander (cilantro)

Remove the peel and pith from the oranges and cut in half. Feed one orange through the juicer, then feed the coriander and then feed the second orange through. Pour into a glass and serve immediately. Enjoy!

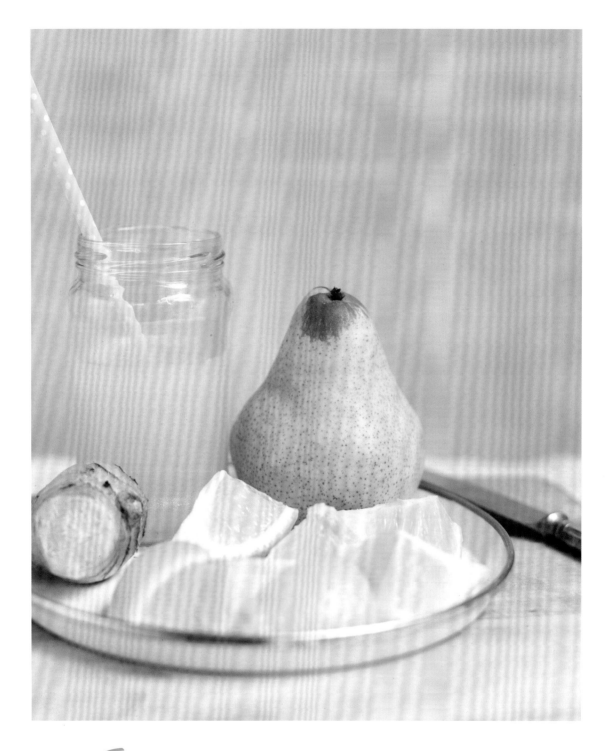

Tip: WHEN JUICING IT IS BEST TO ALWAYS USE FRUIT AND
VEGETABLES IN ORDER FROM SOFT TO HARDER TO ENSURE THEY GET
THROUGH THE JUICER, FOR EXAMPLE KALE BEFORE CUCUMBER.

TURMERIC SHOT

1 knob ginger
1 piece turmeric root
½ lemon
1 pinch cayenne pepper

Feed the ginger, turmeric and lemon through the juicer. Pour into a shot glass. Sprinkle the cayenne over. Serve immediately. Enjoy!

ORANGE FLU AND COLD FIGHTER

1 orange
1 pink grapefruit
1 knob ginger
½ lemon
1 pinch cayenne pepper

Cut the orange and grapefruit in half. Remove the peel and pith from both halves then cut the orange and grapefruit to fit into the juicer. Feed the orange, grapefruit and ginger through the juicer. Pour into a glass. Using your citrus reamer, squeeze the lemon directly into your juice. Sprinkle the cayenne pepper over. Serve immediately. Enjoy!

Tip: IF YOU DON'T LOVE THE GRAPEFRUIT YOU CAN USE ½ GRAPEFRUIT AND 2 ORANGES INSTEAD. FEEL BETTER!

MANDARIN STRAWBERRY JUICE

3 mandarins
5 strawberries
1 lime

Remove the peel from the mandarins and break in half. Hull the strawberries. Feed the mandarins and strawberries through the juicer. Pour into a glass. Using your citrus reamer, squeeze the lime directly into your juice. Serve immediately. Enjoy!

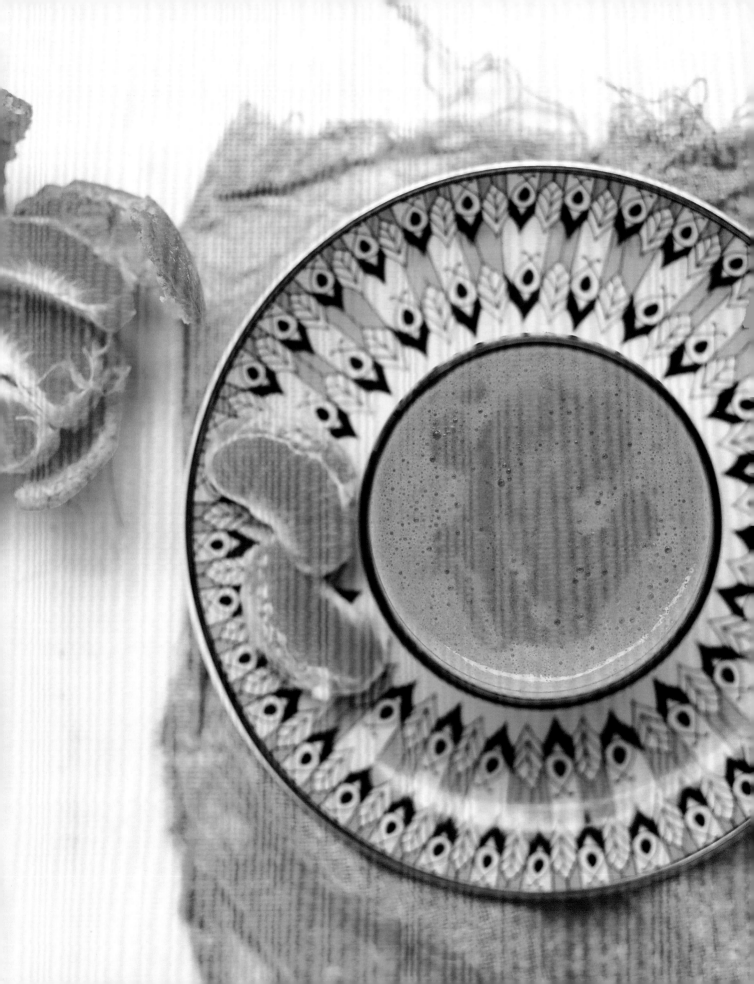

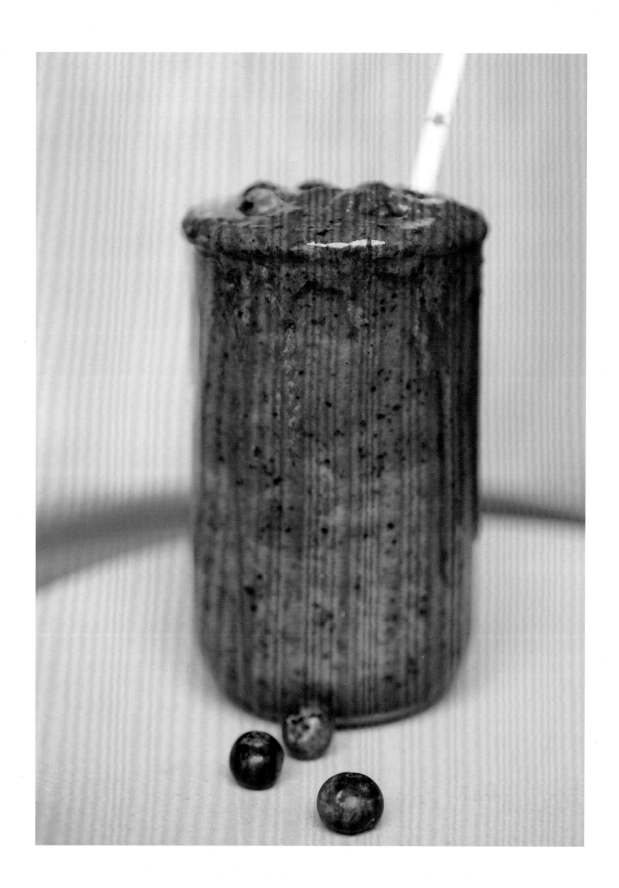

ORANGE ZINGER JUICE

2   carrots
1   grapefruit
2   knobs ginger
1   lemon

Cut the tips off the carrots. Cut the grapefruit in half, then peel and remove the pith, and cut the grapefruit to fit into the juicer. Feed the carrots, grapefruit and ginger through the juicer. Pour into a glass. Using your citrus reamer, squeeze the lemon directly into your juice. Serve immediately. Enjoy!

FULL OF BERRIES SMOOTHIE

1   cup homemade nut milk (see 'Nut Milk – unsweetened' recipe, page 59, and choose hazelnut, macadamia or walnut)
1½ cups berries (blackberries, blueberries and/or raspberries), fresh or preferably frozen
1   tablespoon ABC (almond, Brazil nut, cashew) butter
1   tablespoon cacao nibs
1½ tablespoons goji berries

Add all the ingredients to the blender. Try adding maca powder for an extra boost! Blend and enjoy!

Tip: PLAY AROUND USING DIFFERENT NUT MILKS WITH DIFFERENT BERRIES AND FIND YOUR FAVOURITE-TASTING POWERFUL SMOOTHIE!

WATERMELON AND CARROT SMOOTHIE

2   carrots

1   knob ginger

2   cups chopped watermelon, rind removed

2   cups ice (optional)

Cut the tips off the carrots and chop them in large pieces. Peel the ginger. Add all the ingredients to the blender. Blend and enjoy!

Tip: WHILE I NORMALLY SKIP THE ICE, SOMETIMES WATERMELON WITH ICE TASTES MORE REFRESHING.

HEALTHY ALMOND SMOOTHIE

1   banana, fresh or preferably frozen

1   cup of almond milk (see 'Almond Milk – unsweetened' recipe, page 58)

1   teaspoon almond butter

1   teaspoon hemp seeds

1   teaspoon chlorella or chlorophyll powder

    pinch of cinnamon

Peel the banana and cut in half. Add the banana, almond milk, almond butter, hemp seeds and chlorophyll powder to the blender. Blend. Pour into a glass and add a pinch of cinnamon. Enjoy!

SWEET SPINACH AND KALE SMOOTHIE

1   handful spinach

1   handful kale

1   apple

1   lemon

1   cup coconut water

1   teaspoon spirulina powder

Cut the spinach and kale into pieces. Peel, core and chop the apple. Peel and remove the pith from the lemon. Add the ingredients to a blender. Blend and enjoy!

DRAGON FRUIT AND GREENS SMOOTHIE

2   handfuls spinach
½   dragon fruit (pitaya)
1   cup almond milk (see
    'Almond Milk – unsweetened'
    recipe, page 58)
½   cup blueberries, fresh or
    preferably frozen

Cut the spinach into pieces. Peel the dragon fruit. Add all the ingredients to the blender. Try stirring in 1 teaspoon of spirulina powder, chlorella or wheatgrass to add some vitamins and minerals. Blend and enjoy!

SWEET DRAGON FRUIT SMOOTHIE

1   banana, fresh or preferably
    frozen
½   cup strawberries, fresh or
    frozen
½   dragon fruit (pitaya)
1   cup filtered water

Peel the banana and cut in half. Hull the strawberries. Peel the dragon fruit. Add all the ingredients to the blender. Try adding maca powder to this powerhouse smoothie. Blend and enjoy!

FRUITY COCONUT SMOOTHIE

½   cup mango, fresh or
    preferably frozen
1   small bunch mint
1   cup coconut water
1   cup berries (blackberries,
    blueberries and/or
    raspberries), fresh or
    preferably frozen
1   teaspoon coconut oil

Peel the mango and cut into pieces. Chop the mint. Add all the ingredients to the blender. Try stirring in 1 teaspoon of spirulina powder, chlorella or wheatgrass to add some vitamins and minerals. Blend and enjoy!

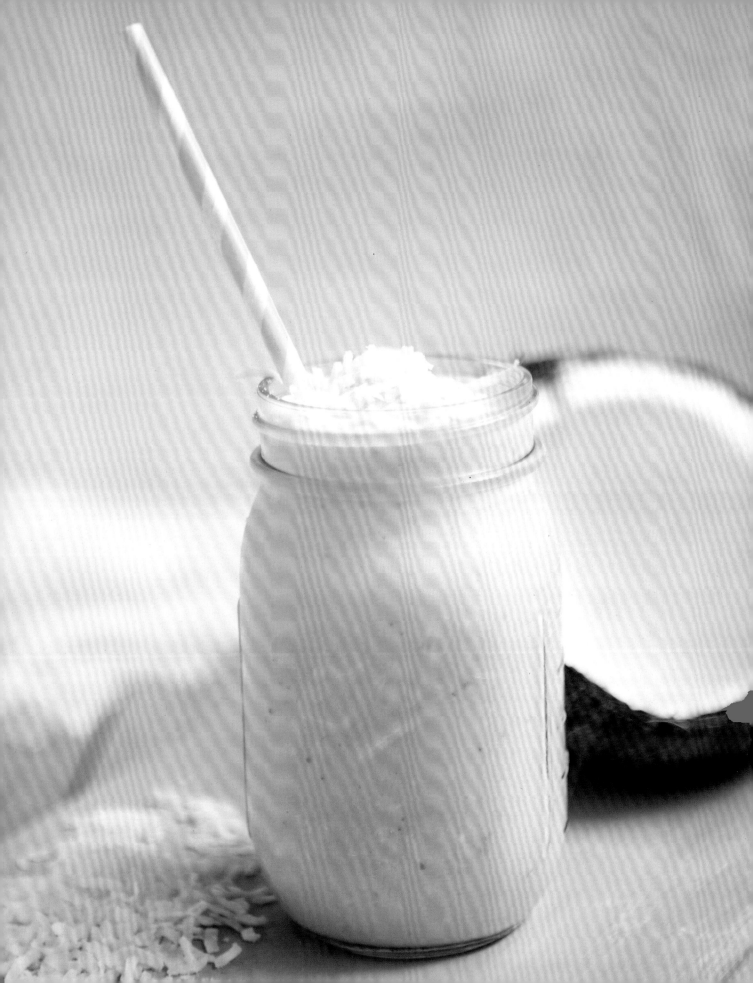

CHAPTER 7

HYDRATE

Are you already juicing and exercising and want to add some extra juicy love to your life? Are you feeling like you just fell off the wagon and want to kick back into a health regime? Or are you getting ready for summer and need to banish the bloat? Well, I have you covered. Here are some fun-loving, butt-kicking, delicious and healthy juices that will get you excited, energized and feeling great.

Stay hydrated with fruit and vegetables that are loaded with water. The best of the bunch are lettuce, watermelon, cucumber, pineapple, blueberries, tomato, celery and grapefruit — delicious and good for you!

TIPS FOR STAYING HYDRATED

Let's look at some powerful fruit and vegetables as well as superfoods that will help you recover from hangovers, power-up after intense exercise and kick you back into gear while being fully hydrated! Here are a few great things to keep in mind when juicing and blending:

» **Add bananas to your smoothies; they are loaded with magnesium and potassium.**

» **Cherries are an anti-inflammatory fruit and really beneficial after a long workout.**

- » Coconut water is loaded with potassium and super hydrating.

- » Load up on leafy greens such as kale and spinach for much-needed vitamins and minerals.

- » Try a vegan protein powder, such as pea or brown rice, which helps keep your muscles working hard.

- » Watermelon is high in water content, to hydrate you.

- » Wheatgrass is loaded with iron, just what you need after a long night or crazy workout.

JUICY RECIPES

BANISH THE BLOAT JUICE

2 cups chopped watermelon, rind removed

1 handful mint

1 knob ginger

Feed all the ingredients through a juicer. Pour into a glass. Serve immediately and enjoy!

WATERMELON AND KALE COOLER JUICE

2 cups chopped watermelon, rind removed

1 handful kale

Feed half the watermelon, then the kale, and then the rest of the watermelon through the juicer. Pour into a glass. Serve immediately and enjoy!

Feel free to try this one in the blender for a thick smoothie option!

WATERMELON HYDRATOR JUICE

2 cups chopped watermelon, rind removed

3 ice cubes

Feed the watermelon through the juicer. Pour into a glass and add ice. Serve immediately and enjoy!

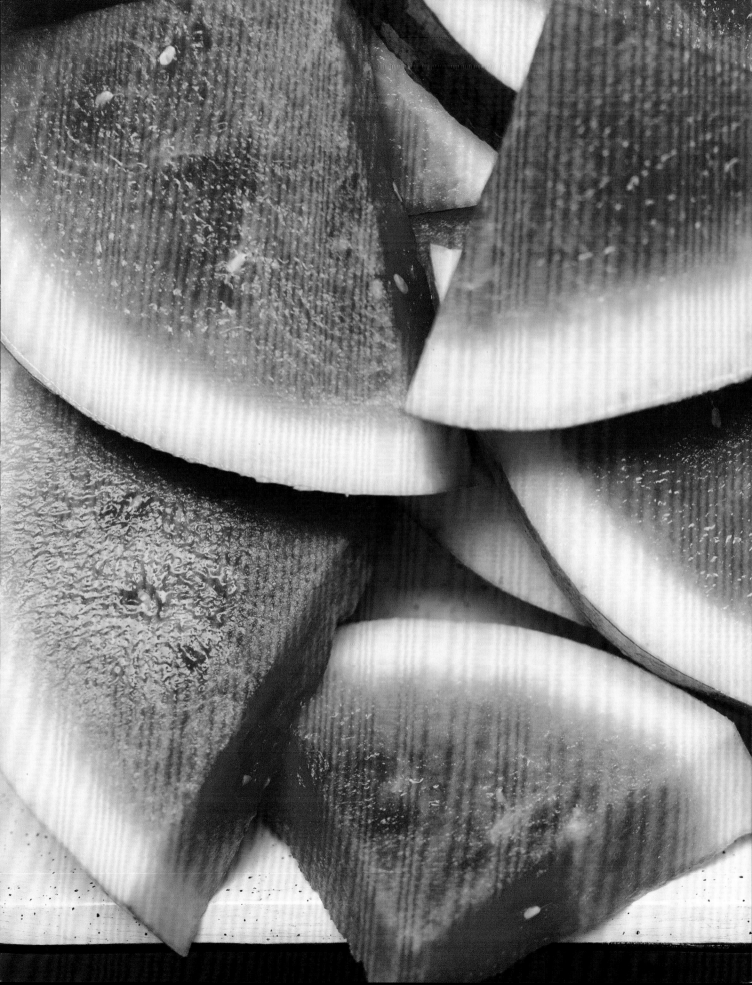

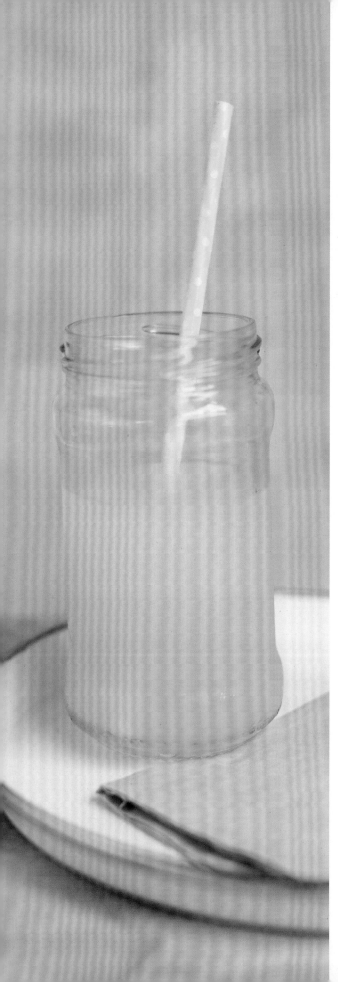

CLEAN APPLE JUICE

 1 apple
 2 handfuls cos (romaine) lettuce
 ¼ cucumber

Cut the apple to fit into the juicer.
Feed the ingredients through the juicer.
Pour into a glass. Serve immediately
and enjoy!

GREEN HYDRATOR JUICE

 2 stalks celery
 1 cucumber
 1 handful kale
 ½ lemon

Feed the celery, cucumber and kale
through the juicer. Pour into a glass.
Using your citrus reamer, squeeze the
lemon directly into your juice. Serve
immediately. Enjoy!

GREEN CORIANDER JUICE

 1 green apple
 2 handfuls spinach
 1 cucumber
 1 small handful mint
 1 small handful coriander
    (cilantro)
 1 knob ginger

Cut the apple to fit into the juicer.
Feed the ingredients through the juicer.
Pour into a glass. Serve immediately.
Enjoy!

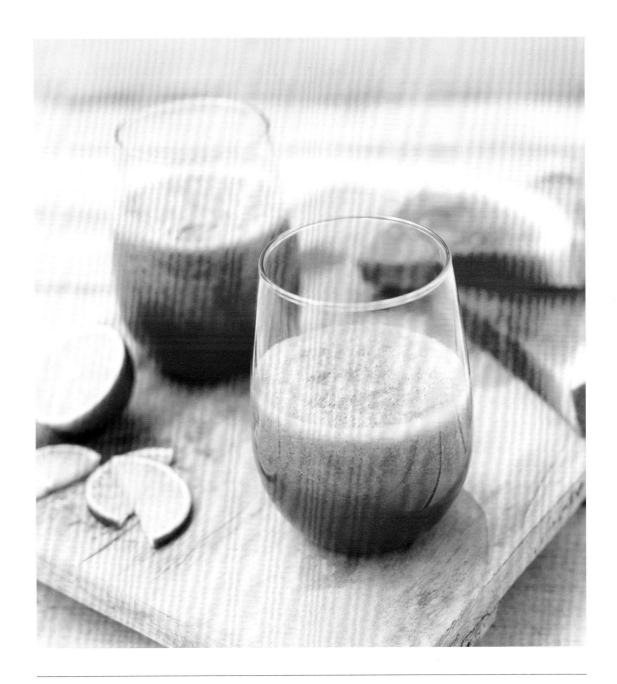

WATERMELON SMOOTHIE

½ lime
1 knob ginger
2 cups chopped watermelon, rind removed
2 cups ice (optional)

Peel and remove the pith from the lime. Peel the ginger. Add all the ingredients to the blender. Blend and enjoy!

CHERRY HYDRATOR SMOOTHIE

3 handfuls cherries, fresh or preferably frozen
1 cup filtered water
2 tablespoons protein powder (pea, brown rice or combination)
1 tablespoon ABC (almond, Brazil nut and cashew) butter

Remove the pits from the cherries. Add all the ingredients to the blender. Blend and enjoy!

COCONUT CHERRY HYDRATOR SMOOTHIE

1 handful cherries, fresh or preferably frozen
1 banana, fresh or preferably frozen
1 cup coconut water
1 teaspoon cacao nibs
1 teaspoon chlorella powder

Remove the pits from the cherries. Peel the banana and cut in half. Add all the ingredients to the blender. Blend and enjoy!

SWEET KALE SMOOTHIE

1 handful kale
½ pineapple
1 banana, fresh or preferably frozen
1 cup coconut water
1 tablespoon protein powder (pea, brown rice or combination)

Cut the kale into pieces. Peel the pineapple and cut into pieces. Peel the banana and cut in half. Add all the ingredients to the blender. Blend and enjoy!

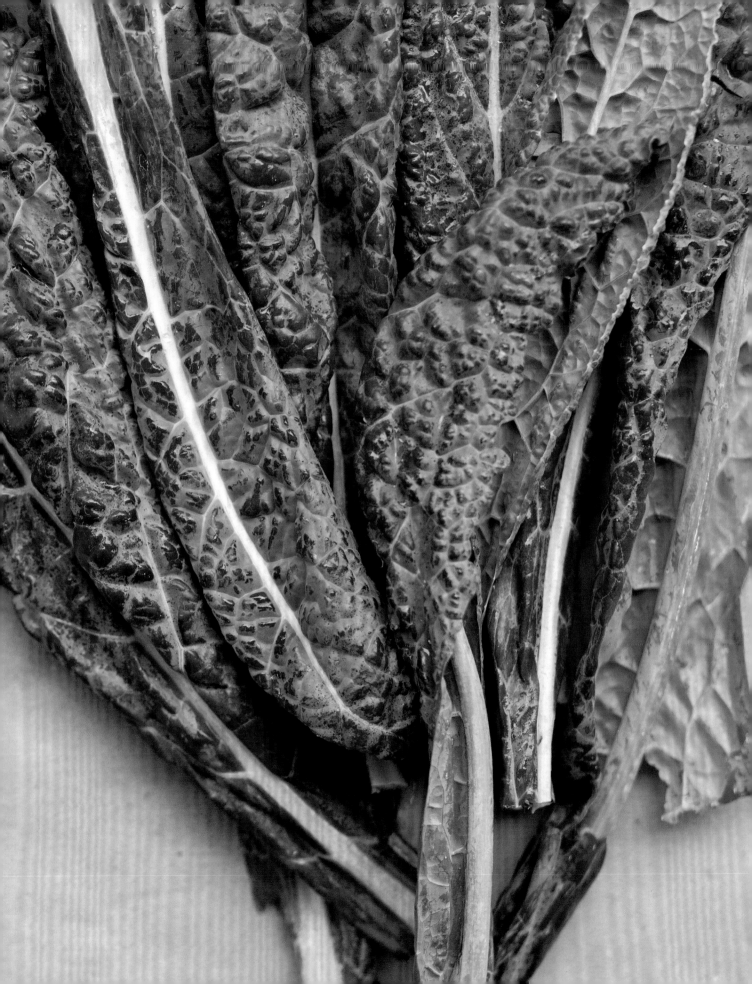

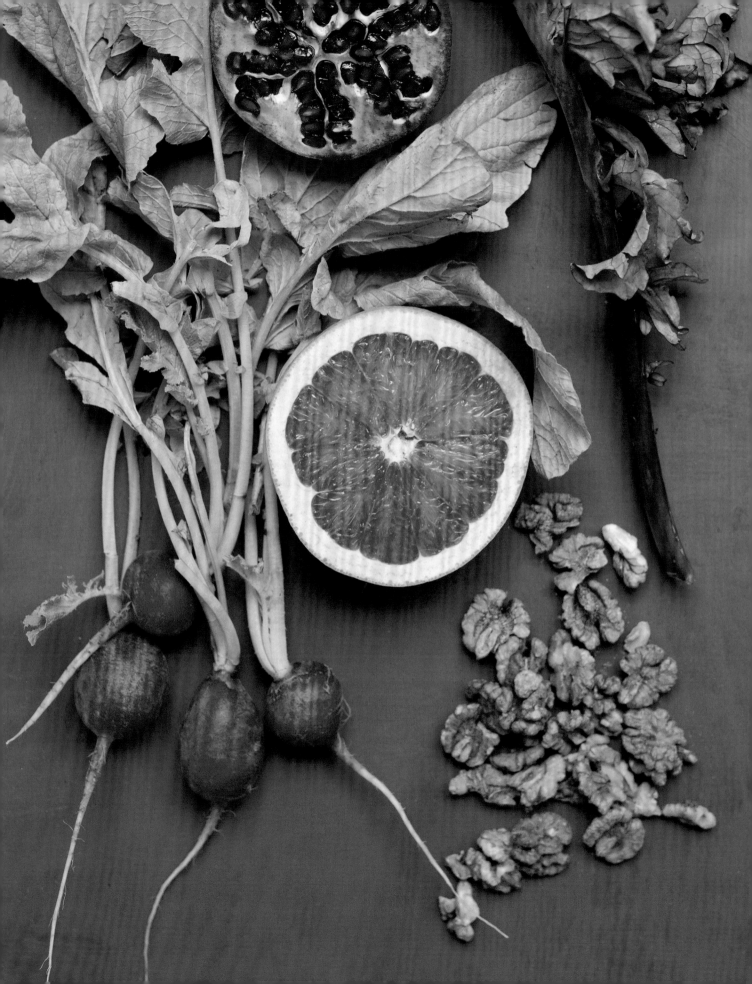

CHAPTER 8

CLEANSE

Heal your body. Heal your mind. As you know, I strongly recommend that you incorporate into your diet at least a daily juice and smoothie filled with vegetables, fruit and superfoods. I also recommend giving your digestive system a break and pumping your system with an overflowing amount of vitamins and minerals through an occasional juice cleanse. These are important to ensure our system is cleansed, alkalized, balanced and prepared for healing. Think of a juice cleanse as cleaning out the toxins to leave room for health!

SO, WHAT IS A JUICE CLEANSE?

A juice cleanse is a way to kick-start your system and get back on track. You can choose either a one-, three- or five-day cleanse. You can include only juices or mix raw food with your juices, depending on how hard-core you want to be. Some people need to chew and want to keep raw food as part of the cleanse, and that is perfectly fine — you should do whatever it takes to keep you on track and avoid the temptation to give up. Do what you think you can. (Remember, though, it is not safe to cleanse or detox if you are pregnant or breastfeeding.)

A cleanse can be the perfect way to reboot and rebalance.

BENEFITS OF A CLEANSE

You will have more energy!
You will glow!
You will feel great!

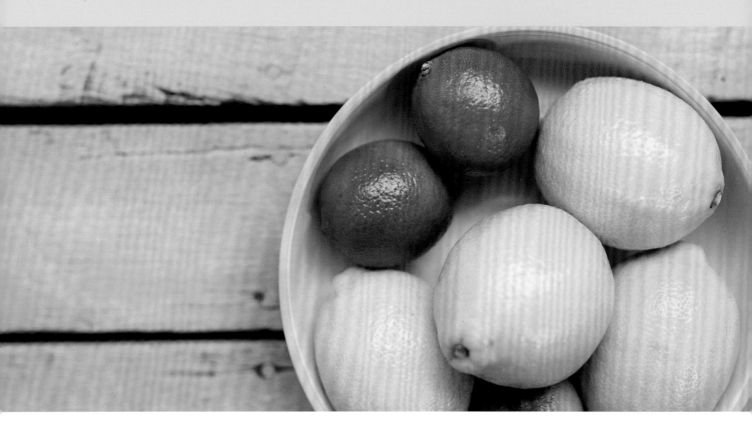

WHY CLEANSE?

There are countless reasons to do a juice cleanse, even if just once a year. Here
is the shortlist:

» **Give your gut a day off! By laying off fibre, your digestive
system can work less. Remember that juicing requires very
little from your digestive system, allowing your digestive tract
to rest and heal.**

» Get your groove back! When you first start the cleanse you might feel exhausted. If you do the three- or five-day cleanse you will see your energy levels drop and then spike up and hit great heights. This doesn't happen as obviously with a shorter cleanse, but it still occurs. However, remember that you won't spike and fall again and again like you do after sweets; you will feel alive and well after the cleanse kick-starts your system.

» Lose weight! If you don't need to lose weight, then lucky you! Juice cleanses banish the bloat, so any water retention starts to shed. Be careful not to dive back into your old habits after the cleanse, otherwise you will put that weight back on.

» Improve your health! You will see a major change in yourself, especially if you do the longer three- or five-day cleanse. You will feel better. You will look better. You will be better.

WHEN TO CLEANSE

Some people do juice cleanses once a year, like cleaning out their summer wardrobe. Some cleanse as the seasons change, others quarterly or even monthly. I don't recommend cleansing more than once a month or more than twelve times a year; nor do I suggest you cleanse for longer than five days.

Try changing your diet to a raw-food diet as part of a pre-cleanse, which will be the prep time before you cleanse. Stick with the raw food post-cleanse to keep the benefits of the cleanse going. It is important to decide how long you want to cleanse for and then plan for at least an extra few days on each end, giving yourself at least a week per cleanse.

CLEANSING TIPS

» Prepare. Prepare. Prepare. I can't say it enough. Don't decide the night before that you want to do a juice cleanse. Think about the cleanse and prepare at least a week or more in advance. Buy all of your ingredients ahead of time and make sure you plan how you will achieve success!

» Plan to pre-cleanse. I always suggest a day or two of a raw diet that includes plant foods, choosing only fruit and vegetables. That means giving up wheat, gluten, dairy, sugar, caffeine and alcohol. Avoid all processed foods.

» Drink plenty of filtered water. Try using an alkaline filter. Water is your best friend and helps flush out the toxins, leaving you feeling good. Squeeze a little lemon in all of your water to makes it alkaline, which will give you added benefits.

» Use only organic fruit and vegetables in your juices, to ensure that you aren't ingesting any of the pesticides you are trying to clear your system of.

» Leave out the fibre. Cleansing is an opportunity for your body to heal, therefore we will leave out the fibre and stick to juices. If you can't live without the fibre, you can do a juice-until-dinner cleanse or a juice-and-raw-food cleanse.

» Take time off social plans. Cleansing and going out with friends is never a good combination. Cleansing is a great time to stay home reading, catching up on sleep, taking long baths and listening to good music. So, skip the parties the week of a cleanse.

» Relax. No exercise this week either. Rest and catch up on sleep. Exercise will be too hard on your body and could have a reverse effect. During a cleanse you will need true rest and an opportunity for your body to repair itself.

» Get a massage! Soak up the oil and the relaxation.

» Take probiotics. Research what might be best for you, but take these every day during the cleanse.

» Drink hot water with lemon every morning; it is incredibly good for you. Simply boil hot water and add a squeeze of fresh lemon juice, then drink up!

» Post-cleanse by sticking with a raw-food diet. Slowly introduce new foods each day and see how your body tolerates them. I find that dairy is really tough on my body; see how it affects you.

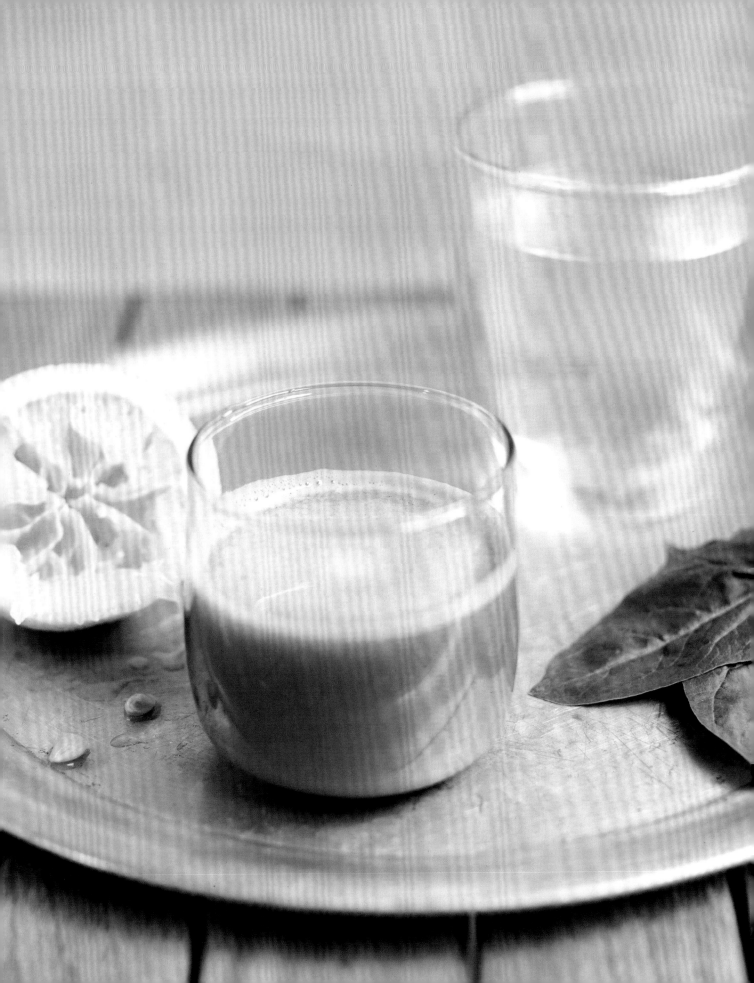

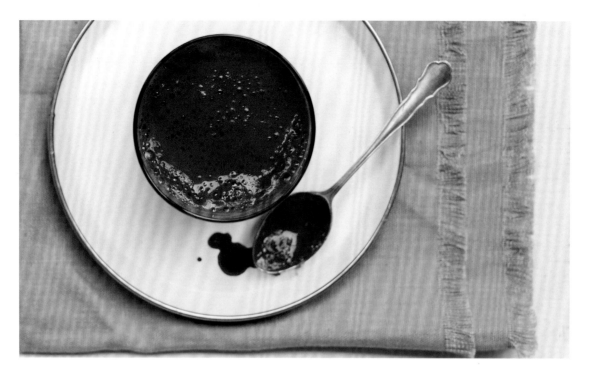

CLEANSING JUICY RECIPES

JUICY 1 - BREAKFAST

1	apple
1	handful kale
3	stalks celery
1	cucumber
1	knob ginger
1	lemon

Cut the apple to fit into the juicer. Feed the apple, kale, celery, cucumber and ginger through the juicer. Pour into a glass. Using your citrus reamer, squeeze the lemon directly into your juice. Serve immediately. Enjoy!

JUICY 2 - SNACK

1	grapefruit
1	handful mint
1	knob ginger

Cut the grapefruit in half, then peel and remove the pith, and cut the grapefruit to fit into the juicer. Feed the grapefruit, mint and ginger through the juicer. Pour into a glass. Serve immediately. Enjoy!

JUICY 3 - LUNCH

1	handful kale
½	cucumber
3	stalks celery
1	handful parsley
1	lemon

Feed the kale, cucumber, celery and parsley through the juicer. Pour into a glass. Using your citrus reamer, squeeze the lemon directly into your juice. Serve immediately. Enjoy!

JUICY 4 - SNACK

1	beet, with greens
1	apple
½	lemon
1	knob ginger

Remove the greens from the beet and set aside. Cut the beet in half to fit into the juicer. Cut the apple to fit into the juicer. Remove the peel and pith from the lemon. Feed the beet, beet greens, apple, ginger and lemon through the juicer. Pour into a glass. Serve immediately. Enjoy!

JUICY 5 - DINNER

This is a shot of extra cleansing love, but if you want to try it as a juice instead of as part of a cleanse, I suggest adding 1 cup of filtered water to the recipe.

1	knob ginger
1	piece turmeric root
½	lemon
1	pinch cayenne pepper

Feed the ginger, turmeric and lemon through the juicer. Pour into a shot glass. Sprinkle the cayenne over. Serve immediately. Enjoy!
Note: If you are looking for this drink to last, pour in 1 cup of filtered water and stir.

NUT MILK - DESSERT

See 'Nut Milk — unsweetened' recipe, page 59. Choose almond or cashew milk. Not a fan of nut milk? No problem, try coconut milk instead. See 'Coconut milk' recipe, page 60.

THE TOP 10 ESSENTIALS

REMEMBER THESE TOP TIPS WHENEVER YOU'RE JUICING AND BLENDING!

1. The main difference between juicing and blending is that juicing separates the juice from the fibre while blending keeps the fibre intact.

2. Juicing uses a centrifugal or slow-masticating juicer while blending or smoothie-making uses a blender.

3. Wash all vegetables and fruit whether juicing or blending.

4. Prep your ingredients ahead of time and freeze the fruit you want to use in smoothies.

5. Use organic produce when you can, or use the Dirty Dozen list as your guide (see page 20) to buying organic fruit and vegetables.

6. Start your day off with water and lemon to keep the body alkaline.

7. Change up your vegetables; don't have the same greens every day.

8. Stick to three vegetables and one fruit in juices to keep your glycemic levels low.

9. Try a juice cleanse as seasons change.

10. Juice every single day!

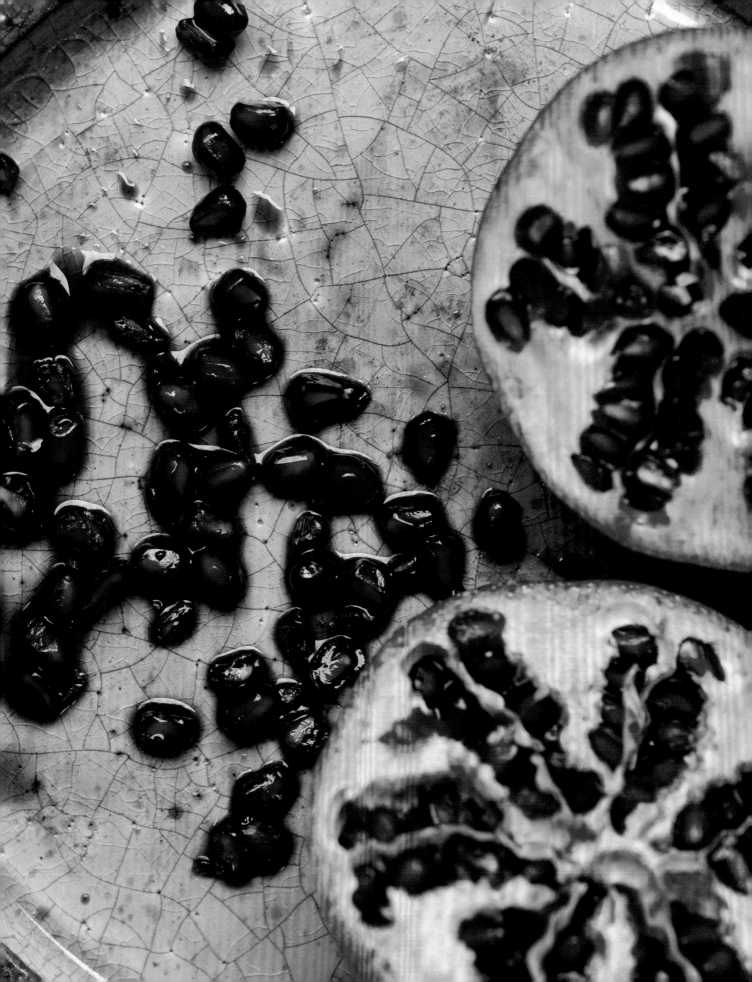

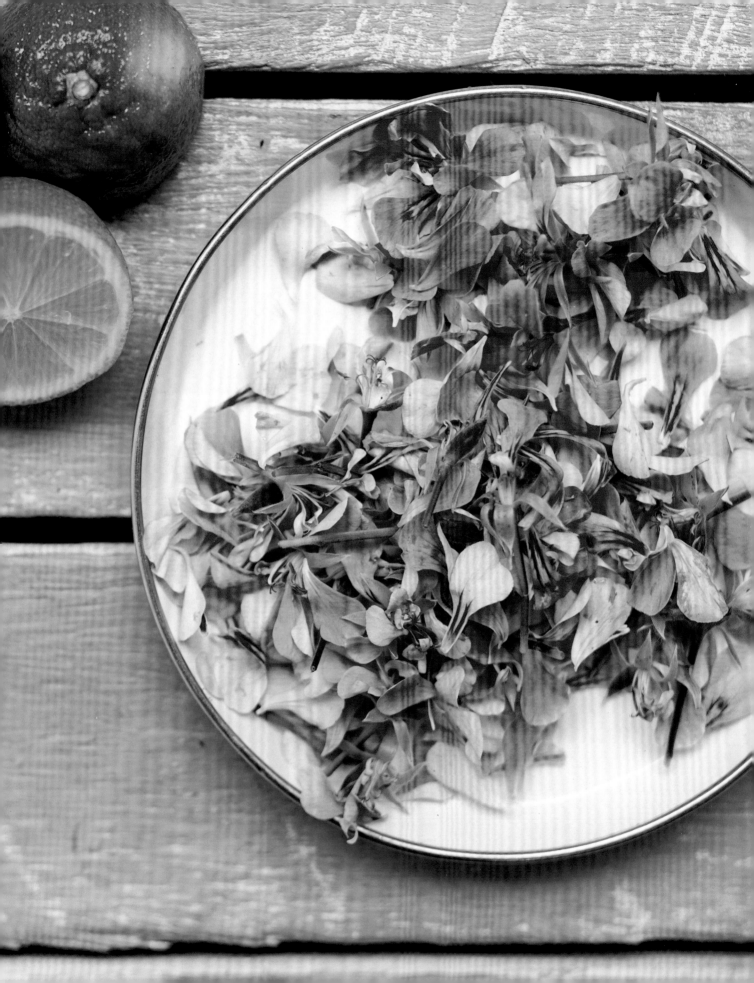

THANK YOU FROM THE BOTTOM OF MY HEART

To all the beautiful people in my life who have supported me, made this world a better place for me and encouraged me time and time again. Your encouragement, love and ongoing support helped to create this book, for without your wisdom and support this book wouldn't have been complete. So, much love and thanks to you.

Benny Thomas, for believing in me and making this book happen.

Gareth Thomas, so much gratitude for taking a chance on me.

Anouska Jones, the dream publisher to work with, who is supportive and always positive.

Claire de Medici, my editor, for your patience and understanding and being a wonderful editor.

Bayleigh Vedegalo, my absolutely amazing photographer, you are not only talented, but a pleasure to work with. These images are magic because of you.

Helen Ridge, thank you for giving your stamp of approval on pieces of this book and encouraging me to look after my health.

Suzanne Price, the true juice guru. Thank you for all you taught me.

Paula Tursi, for the life-long love and support. For helping me create the life I have today.

Daisy Meyers, thank you for all the wellness tips and ensuring that I quickly adapted to the wellness culture in Australia.

Mom and Dad, thank you for a lifetime of love and support. For always encouraging and believing I could do anything I put my mind to.

Max, my juice lab rat! Thank you for testing all of my juices, giving honest and loving feedback. I couldn't have created this book without you.

Indi, thank you for inspiring me every single day. From the moment you were conceived until the moment you were born we created this book together.

Joe, my husband, soul mate and love of my life — thank you. Thank you for believing in everything I do. For all your love and support. For always being a fan of our juicy lifestyle, trying my juices and going along with all my wacky ways!

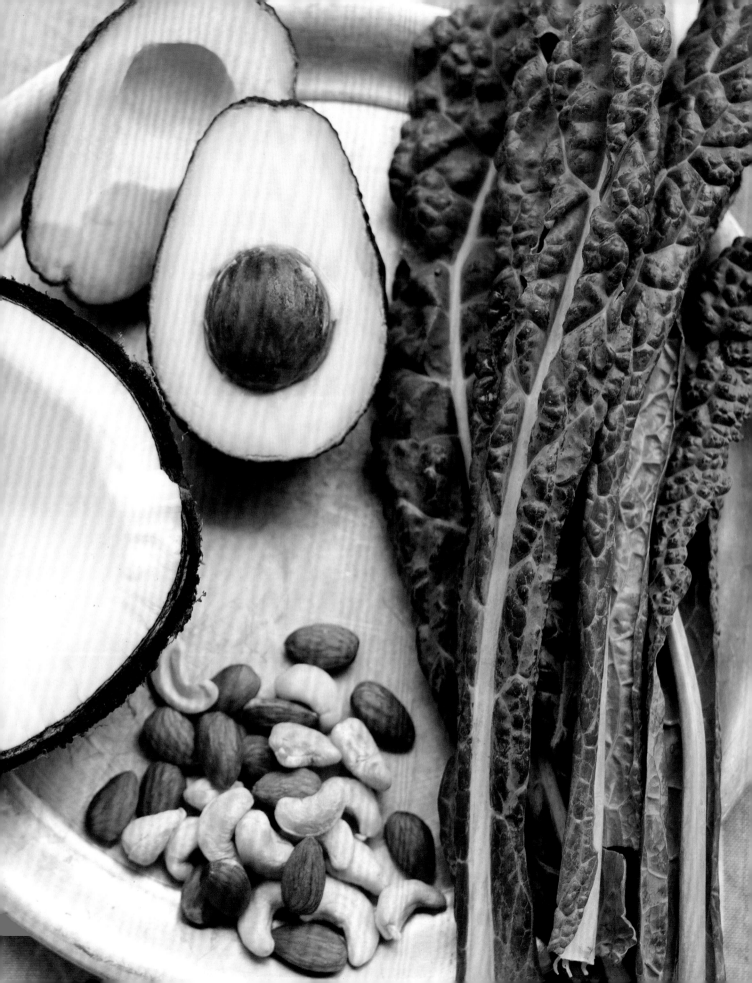

GENERAL INDEX

RECIPE INDEX